Action Evaluation of Health Programmes and Changes

A handbook for a user-focused approach

John Øvretveit

Foreword by Chris Ham

RADCLIFFE MEDICAL PRESS

Radcliffe Medical Press Ltd
18 Marcham Road
Abingdon
Oxon OX14 1AA
United Kingdom

www.radcliffe-oxford.com
The Radcliffe Medical Press electronic catalogue and online ordering facility.
Direct sales to anywhere in the world.

British Library Cataloguing in Publication Data

A catalogue record for this book is available from the British Library.

ISBN 1 85775 925 7

Typeset by Joshua Associates Ltd, Oxford
Printed and bound by TJ International Ltd, Padstow, Cornwall

Contents

Foreword

John Øvretveit has written a clear and practical introduction to evaluation in health services. Drawing on his experience as a researcher and teacher, Øvretveit focuses particularly on evaluations intended to influence policy and practice. In a wide-ranging review, he explains how evaluations are conducted, reviews the tools available to evaluators, and discusses the political and ethical dilemmas that may arise.

The great virtue of Øvretveit's approach is that it is simple without being simplistic. Øvretveit recognises both the opportunities available to evaluators and the obstacles they may encounter along the way. The book will therefore be a valuable introduction for evaluators and those involved in commissioning evaluations.

As its subtitle indicates, *Action Evaluation of Health Programmes and Changes* is a handbook that takes the reader on a step-by-step guide through the field. It will be of particular interest to those involved in evaluations in which experimental designs are not feasible and where alternative methods have to be adopted. Øvretveit helpfully sets out the strengths and weaknesses of different approaches and includes in the text a series of practical tips based on his experience. At a time when 'evidence based everything' is high on the agenda, his introduction to user focused evaluation will be welcomed by researchers and practitioners.

Chris Ham
Health Services Management Centre
University of Birmingham
October 2001

Preface

The need for evaluation in healthcare has never been greater, yet the evaluation methods used often do not provide the evidence which decision makers need. Action evaluation focuses on the evaluation user's needs and designs the evaluation to answer their questions within the resources and time available. The approach can be used to maximise the usefulness of an evaluation carried out using either traditional methods or methods less well known in healthcare.

This book describes this 'user-focused' action evaluation approach for evaluating health programmes, policies and changes. It shows that evidence for making decisions about these interventions can be gathered using a broader range of methods than is usually recognised in healthcare. In asking 'evaluation for whom and for what?', the book defines validity of evidence in relation to usefulness as well as in terms of whether systematic methods were followed.

Managers, practitioners, policy makers, researchers and students will find this a practical book on evaluation which gives a broad view of the approaches needed. It gives tools to make sense of an evaluation quickly, as well as guidance for carrying one out, and for ensuring that evaluators gather evidence which can be used for making better informed decisions.

John Øvretveit
October 2001

About the author

Dr John Øvretveit is an experienced evaluator of change and teacher of both social science and medical research evaluation methods. He is Professor of Health Policy and Management at the Nordic School of Public Health in Gothenberg, the School of Medicine, University of Bergen, and the Karolinska Institute, Stockholm.

Chapter 1

Action evaluation: what is it and why evaluate?

We judge the value of things all the time. But we are not usually aware of the criteria we are using or on which evidence we base our judgements. Evaluation ideas and evaluations help us to make better judgements and our actions more effective.

Evaluation literacy, like computer literacy, is now a work requirement in healthcare, even for politicians. The question is not whether we should evaluate, but how well we do it. There are many different methods we could use. The best method is the one which answers the evaluation user's questions using their values – given the time and money available.

Introduction

This book is for professionals working in healthcare and policy makers. It has a practical 'how to' orientation, which comes from my own experience of making evaluations and teaching colleagues how to use and carry out evaluations. It gives tools for planning and carrying out an evaluation and for understanding and assessing one. It describes an action evaluation approach as well as providing an introduction to other approaches for evaluating health activities, programmes and change.

Much has been written about treatment evaluation, but there is less which is of practical use about how to evaluate a health programme, a change or any activity which people are carrying out. In healthcare we tend to apply a medical research approach to evaluate everything and assume that valid evidence can only come from carefully controlled experimental trials. Sometimes these methods are appropriate, but often they are neither possible nor give the necessary answers within a reasonable time when we need to evaluate health programmes and change.

This book aims to show the range of methods which can be used for evaluating the many different non-treatment activities, changes, policies and other 'things' or 'interventions' which we need to evaluate in healthcare. It aims to show how an action evaluation approach can maximise the usefulness of an evaluation carried out using traditional or less conventional methods. It offers a broad conception of 'evidence' in answering the question: 'Evaluation for whom and for what?'

Evaluation has now become a part of everyday life in healthcare. As health professionals, we monitor our patient's response to a treatment and have an ethical obligation and professional duty to evaluate our own practice. As managers and policy makers, we need to ensure that resources are used to the best effect and that we can explain to the public why we have made certain choices on their behalf. This is a public of consumers who are increasingly using the findings from health evaluations to challenge decisions, a public of taxpayers who want to know that democratic decisions were implemented and that money was well spent on the latest reform or hospital merger. We all need to use evaluation principles and methods to improve our practice and services, as well as to avoid expensive mistakes in health policies or reforms.

Health evaluation raises questions about our own and others' values and about what we consider important in life. It involves questions about how we change clinical and managerial practice and about how governments and organisations make health policies which affect us all. We will see how evaluations are used to advance and defend powerful interests and how the evaluator has to continually choose between the ideal and the practical. We will see how simple evaluation methods are breaking the division between research and practice, how more practitioners are applying the methods to reorganise the way they give care and how managers and politicians are increasingly using evaluations in making decisions.

Box 1.1: This book:
- describes how health personnel can use and carry out an evaluation, as well as how external researchers can make evaluations
- considers methods to evaluate any activity or change: a healthcare service, a health promotion programme, a change to a health organisation, a policy or a healthcare reform
- views evaluation as a service to a customer and proposes an action evaluation approach which is 'user focused'

- describes different evaluation methods, which are suited to different subjects and evaluation users
- views evaluation as an integral part of professional practice and of a service's programme for continuous improvement and clinical governance.

Learning about and using evaluations contributes to our professional development – we develop skills which are immediately useful in our everyday work – but also to our personal development. Evaluation makes us think about our values and the values of other people: how should we or others judge the value of a health programme or a change? Is efficiency the only criterion by which to value it? How would we know if something we value has been achieved? How do we judge the value of the effects of a change on patients, carers and professionals? What is really important to us and to them? If you are asking questions about what is really important in your own personal and professional life and what is worth spending time on, then evaluation provides some tools to help think the issues through.

Ideas about evaluation are not difficult but are sometimes presented in confusing ways. This is because there are different views about the boundaries between evaluation, research, quality assurance and everyday professional practice. It is also because there are different scientific paradigms in evaluation and strongly held views about what is to be counted as evidence. Each of these different approaches is often presented as the only true way and the existence and value of other approaches ignored. This book takes the view that every approach is the best way – in the right circumstances. It also presents a practical action evaluation approach to put evaluation more in the hands of ordinary people working in and using healthcare.

The dominant paradigm in healthcare is the experimental medical research paradigm: certain knowledge only comes from treating the 'thing' or action to be evaluated as an experiment. The evaluator should plan the evaluation and how to gather objective data before and after the action is carried out on people or organisations. They should be objective and detached. Another approach is to evaluate something after it has happened by asking people for their judgements and to increase the validity of the picture built from asking many different people using a variety of social science methods.

This book describes both these approaches and others. This is because, in healthcare, we need to be able to choose the evaluation approach which is most suited to the type of intervention we are evaluating and to the informational needs of the users of the evaluation. The medical research approach to evaluation is not the only approach and health personnel and policy makers need to become more familiar with and use other ways of judging the value of interventions and changes. Lack of familiarity with these methods and the dominant medical research paradigm explain in part why few evaluations are carried out of the many non-treatment interventions and changes which need to be evaluated in healthcare. Evidence-based healthcare needs to include decisions about policies and changes as well as evidence from a variety of methods.

Action evaluation for evaluating health programmes and changes

The first aim of the book is to present evaluation and demonstrate evaluation 'tools' which you can use in everyday work. These tools are methods, concepts and guidance on steps to follow. Methods for evaluating the following types of 'non-treatment interventions', actions and changes are given.

- A specific health service, such as one for depressed older people living at home.
- Health programmes, such as a primary care programme made up of many specific services or a health promotion programme encouraging healthy eating and exercise.
- Methods or models of care organisation such as case management or a new form of team organisation.
- Policies, such as a health policy to reduce cancer or a healthcare policy to prioritise waiting lists or to encourage hospitals and primary care providers to form provider networks.
- Changes to organisations or interventions such as a training pro- gramme or a new method for financing hospitals, the larger changes being called 'reforms'.

The book refers to these 'non-treatment interventions' as programmes and changes. Reforms are changes to how organisations work or relate to each other and can be large scale, such as a national health reform, or small scale, such as a local reform to the structure of one hospital.

Many of these types of interventions or changes to healthcare services are difficult to evaluate using traditional medical research methods, although ingenious ways have been found to use randomisation and controls to evaluate some. The book draws on traditional medical research approaches, but also shows how social scientific methods often better answer the questions of those who want the evaluation (the primary evaluation 'users') even though these methods are less well known in the health sector.

The second aim of this book is to describe an action evaluation approach. What is action evaluation and why is it needed in healthcare? The term 'action evaluation' conveys the idea that evaluation is for action – for the evaluation user to make more informed decisions about what to do in the future. It also conveys the idea that making the evaluation itself is active and carried out in a shorter time than is usual for a conventional research evaluation.

***

Action evaluation – definition

Action evaluation is carried out for one user group, using their value criteria, and provides them with data to make more informed decisions. The evaluator works with the evaluation user to clarify the criteria to be used to judge the value of an intervention, as well as to clarify the decisions which the user has to make which can be informed by the evaluation. Action evaluation collects data about the intervention and its effects and uses comparison to help users to judge value and decide future action. It is collaborative, usually gathers people's subjective perceptions, is carried out in a short time and provides actionable data for evaluation users, but the findings may be less generalisable and less certain than those arising from a conventional research evaluation.

***

Why is action evaluation needed in healthcare? The main reason is the limitations of traditional research evaluation methods when applied to evaluating changes or new programmes which are not as specific and controllable as medical treatments. Often experimental methods and controls cannot be used to evaluate health programmes which change over time or health policies which are difficult to define or to evaluate changes where it is not clear exactly what was changed. Many non-treatment interventions themselves change, are affected by surrounding factors which cannot be controlled and have many short- and long-term outcomes which may be difficult to measure.

Evaluations decision makers – managers, professionals, politicians and patients – need rapid and relevant evaluations of things other than treatments. They need information to help decide whether to stop or continue an activity, a change or a new programme or about how to adjust it to make it more effective. They often do not have time to wait for a research evaluation of a health reform or a policy or a new model of care. Traditional evaluations take a long time to complete, are expensive and often do not give the information which evaluation users need.

This does not mean that detailed research evaluations are not necessary. When they can be done, these evaluations can give more certain information about short- and long-term outcomes and about how the intervention works. Action evaluations are more relevant and useable, but may be less certain and have to state their limitations carefully. Action evaluations can be carried out by service providers themselves, for example in quality improvement or to project manage the implementation of a change.

An action evaluation:

- is designed to give an evaluation 'user' or 'customer' evidence which helps them to make more informed decisions about what they should do, at the time that they need it
- is designed for one user and uses their criteria of valuation to decide which evidence to collect
- collaborates with the evaluation user to clarify why they want the evaluation, their questions about the intervention and outcomes, which decisions the evaluation is to inform and which criteria to use to judge the value of the intervention
- decides the design and data gathering which best meet the needs of the user within the timescale and resources available for the evaluation
- collects people's subjective perceptions about outcomes and about the process of the action or intervention, as well as documentary, statistical, measurement and observational data where this is possible
- uses qualitative data collection and analysis techniques to maximise the validity and reliability of people's subjective reports
- collaborates with service providers or those implementing a change in different ways
- sometimes reports emerging findings during the evaluation (which may change the action or intervention whilst it is being evaluated).

Does this mean that an action evaluation concentrates on one user's questions and ignores the perceptions of the other stakeholders with an interest in a health programme or change? Yes and no. Yes, you have to focus on one user's decision information needs and understand their value criteria and questions if you are to deliver an evaluation which can be used to inform real decisions. Even with unlimited time and money, trying to answer many users' questions will make the evaluation inconclusive and ultimately useless for any one user's decisions.

The negative answer is that the evaluation does not ignore the perceptions which different groups have about the thing you are evaluating and does gather data from different perspectives. The reason is that for the user to make informed decisions, they need to know what different parties think about a health programme or a change. We can find out some effects of a programme or change without looking at what people think, by making objective measures or using statistics. But to value and explain a health programme and change we usually need to understand different people's perceptions. What people think is the outcome *is* an outcome. What people think about a programme or change to which they are exposed can influence what happens.

Action evaluation aims to make evaluation more useful by:

- involving the people who need to make decisions about the thing you are evaluating (the evaluation users) in the process of planning an evaluation
- collecting information which is relevant to people's real values and decisions
- limiting the design of the evaluation to what is needed to answer the questions of one user group and to inform their decisions, hence reducing the time and cost.

> *Evaluations are worse than useless if they are not used, because they take time and money away from other activities.*

There are two reasons for presenting this 'user-focused' approach to action evaluation. First, for simplicity: to demonstrate that evaluation need not be complicated and to provide a simple practical approach for any type of evaluation. Second, to contribute to making evaluations more useful: to make it more likely that the evaluation will be used to change what people do or the decisions they make. Many evaluations are made by people who use their own criteria to judge the value of something and to answer questions which are important to them. Then they complain that decision makers do not take any notice of their evaluation.

The aim of many evaluations is to find out if an intervention or action makes a difference. For example, does a new clinic for diabetic patients make a difference to local people with this health condition? Or does a new work policy make it easier to keep and recruit nurses? We can judge the value of the action by examining the size and type of the difference which the action makes. A new work policy could have many effects, but do we concentrate on investigating the differences which are important for future action? When we choose which data or measures to collect about outcome, is our choice clearly and directly linked to what would help people make decisions about what they should do? Are we even aware what these decisions are? Or do we choose which outcomes to measure because we have a good measuring method or because these outcomes are of interest to us as evaluators?

Evaluation on its own is of no value. An evaluation is only effective when it is used to decide what to do, such as how to change something – our practice, a service or a policy. For example, whether to keep or change the new work policy to ensure we attract and keep scarce nurses. The user-focused approach shows how evaluation can be linked to action so that our decisions, practice and health policies can be better informed. It shows how to concentrate on the evaluation users' informational needs and their value criteria, so as to make the evaluation more useful to them.

> There is nothing wrong with judging the value of something – it is essential to do so. But we can make better decisions if we are clear about which values we are using to make the judgements and have good evidence.

More health workers are carrying out self-evaluation, individually or in groups, often as part of quality assurance. As professional practitioners we need to find out what people value about our service and how well we are performing. We can also assess the effectiveness of a new method which we have started using. We may join with others and use peer review methods to evaluate our service or a change to organisation. The concepts and methods in the book can be used to plan and carry out a valid self-evaluation, as well as to carry out an independent research evaluation of a service, a policy or some other activity.

What is the use of evaluation and why do health professionals and policy makers need to become evaluation literate? The later part of this chapter continues the discussion just begun to give a fuller answer to this question. It explains the difference between evaluation, pure research and quality assurance. First, there is a general overview of the three parts of the book which follow this introductory chapter

Outline of the book

There are three parts to the book: how to make an evaluation; tools for evaluation; and specific subjects. The first part shows how to plan and carry out an evaluation. In doing so it introduces the concepts and methods of evaluation using examples. This first part may be sufficient for some readers, but those who wish to know more will look at Part 2 which discusses concepts and designs and gives a tool for assessing an evaluation. Part 3 then considers specific subjects in more detail.

Learning by doing is the best way for many people. Chapter 2 starts immediately with practical guidance on how to evaluate a health service or programme. Health reforms are different because they aim to change how healthcare functions rather than acting directly on patients, which is what services and many programmes do. Chapter 3 gives guidance on how to evaluate reforms or changes to organisation. Both these chapters introduce the basic tools of evaluation as part of the discussion of how to do an evaluation and through practical examples, rather than presenting these tools in the abstract.

Evaluations are worse than useless if they are not used, because they take time and money away from other activities. Carrying out an evaluation feasibility assessment helps the evaluator and sponsor to decide what they want to evaluate and to avoid an expensive evaluation which is not valid. Chapter 4 describes how to do this, before going on to give tools for planning most types of evaluation. Starting an evaluation is the most difficult time in carrying one out. There are so many choices and different people want different information. The key question is how to limit the evaluation to something which is achievable and useful. The two tools described in Chapter 4 show how to do this: the 'quick guide' and the 'nine questions' guide.

Technical knowledge is not enough to perform a successful evaluation. Evaluators need to expect the unexpected and have strategies to deal with common problems, such as lack of reliable service statistics, lost records and changing timescales. Chapter 5 gives advice about this, as well as how to minimise other problems which often occur, such as 'wobbly interventions' and 'the police car effect'. Problem prevention is also possible by agreeing the roles of the evaluator and other parties during each of the phases of an evaluation described in the chapter.

Part 2 describes in more detail the tools and principles for quickly understanding an evaluation which were used in Part 1. One reason we do not make more use of evaluations in our everyday work is that it takes time to understand and assess an evaluation. Chapters 6 and 7 give the concepts and diagrams for quickly making sense of an evaluation. These concepts and diagrams are simple but powerful methods for assessing and planning an evaluation. They have proven their worth in guiding evaluations of different types and in many teaching programmes. Chapter 6 describes concepts for understanding an evaluation, such as the intervention, the target, value criteria and outcomes, and shows how to draw a summary diagram of an evaluation.

In healthcare we need to evaluate many different types of actions and there are many different users who may want different information.

Therefore we need to be able to use different methods, a subject discussed in Chapter 7, which introduces the six evaluation designs. A process evaluation looks at how an intervention is carried out, such as what people do when they provide a health programme or how a reform is implemented. Two designs for process evaluation are described in Chapter 8. Outcome evaluations look at the difference an intervention makes to the people it is intended for. The before–after difference is the simplest, which is one of the three designs described in Chapter 9.

How do you know if an evaluation you are reading is a good one? This is a question which the evidence-based healthcare movement has answered for treatment evaluations (Gray, 1997). The hierarchy of evidence method for assessing evaluations proposed by this movement is neither valid nor useful for assessing many programme, policy or reform evaluations. Chapter 10 presents an alternative general purpose method which is used for assessing an evaluation to decide whether to act on the findings. It also gives the preparation questions to ask when planning an evaluation and for deciding which design to use.

The last part of the book considers certain subjects in more detail. The book does not discuss data-gathering tools and analysis methods for evaluation in detail because many of the methods for collecting data are the same as those used in other types of research and are well described elsewhere. Chapter 11 gives an overview of the five categories of data-gathering methods and references to other texts on the subject.

Chapter 12 shows how evaluation ethics helps to avoid the problems described in Chapter 5. Ethics gives practical solutions to the many conflicts faced by evaluators and, where solutions are not possible, ethics helps to manage the dilemmas. The chapter also sensitises the evaluator to the politics of evaluation – who gains and who loses from the evaluation – and how this affects the way we carry out an evaluation.

Evaluation and quality assurance are subjects which overlap. Chapter 13 describes how quality assurance can use evaluation research and also how evaluation is an integral part of quality assurance. It shows different ways to evaluate quality and qualefficiency, the latter being the quality performance of a service relative to the resources available to that service.

Chapter 14 discusses what we mean by evidence and facts and different paradigms in evaluation – the positivist and phenomenological. It shows how these paradigms underlie different approaches to evaluation and describes the five main evaluation approaches: the experimental, the economic, the social research, the action evaluation and the managerial approaches. The appendices give definitions and data-gathering tools.

Why evaluate?

Change is now constant in healthcare, but not all changes make things better for patients, health personnel or the population's health. During a stay at my local hospital in Goteborg after I was bitten by a dog when out jogging, I learned that the hospital was to be merged with two others to form a 2850-bed hospital. The newspapers said that it was thought that the merger would reduce costs due to economies of scale and improve quality as a result of increased patient volume for many specialties. But evaluations of mergers elsewhere have found that, above 400–600 beds, average costs increase (Aletras *et al.*, 1997). For some specialties there is an association between quality and volume of patients, but for many this levels off after a relatively low volume is reached. It is thought that for many specialties there is no association, if case mix and prognosis are considered (Posnett, 1999). In Sweden we pay taxes to our local authority, which runs healthcare, and the taxes are high. I noticed that the savings did not materialise and there is now discussion of a 'de-merger' – to save costs and because of the poor employee morale which was attributed to the merger.

The point of this example? How much money could have been saved and dissatisfaction avoided if evaluations of similar mergers elsewhere had been studied? Would the decision have been different? Possibly not, but it would have been more informed. In the future decisions will need to take into account this sort of evidence, rather than being made on purely political grounds. Evaluation also ensures that those making changes are held accountable and pay more attention to the consequences which are likely to follow from their decisions.

Box 1.2: Who makes evaluations?

External evaluators: researchers or consultancy units not directly managed by the sponsor and user of the evaluation

Internal evaluators: units or researchers who are internal to the organisation, who evaluate treatments, services or policies carried out by the organisation or one of its divisions

Practitioner self-evaluation: practitioners or teams who evaluate their own practice so as to improve it.

Box 1.3: Why make evaluations?

- To find out if an action makes a difference (does it work?)
- To find out if the difference is worth the cost (what is the cost-effectiveness or value for money?)
- To improve the service (to get better results, to use fewer resources)
- To check if people have done what they are supposed to do (management accountability and to ensure that democratically decided actions are implemented)

What is evaluation?

Evaluation is judging the value of something by gathering valid information about it in a systematic way and by making a comparison. The purpose of evaluation is to help the user of the evaluation to decide what to do, or to contribute to scientific knowledge.

The first feature of evaluation in this definition is that it is a service for a user. It is this practical orientation which distinguishes evaluation from pure research. Evaluations are carried out for specific users or customers to meet their needs for information for the decisions which they need to make. Clinicians and patients use evaluations of medical treatments to make better informed treatment decisions. An example is an evaluation of a new drug treatment for influenza: should I prescribe this for any of my patients? Policy makers and purchasers also use these evaluations to make decisions about whether to finance certain treatments: are the benefits of the treatment worth the costs? In this book we consider evaluations of health services, programmes, policies and changes to organisation or reforms. The users of these evaluations include clinicians as well as managers and policy makers. They use evaluations to make better informed decisions about how to manage and organise services or whether to implement or adjust health policies and reforms.

The definition also emphasises that evaluation is for action – people do something differently as a result of the knowledge which comes from the evaluation. Later chapters consider how to ensure that an evaluation does lead to action, but we note here that designing the evaluation for and with a specific user increases the chances of this happening.

Evaluation is different from pure scientific research, where there is a more general user and the aim is to contribute to knowledge and not to immediate practical action. However, some evaluations, such as well

Table 1.1: Evaluation is one type of research

	Pure research	Research evaluation	Action evaluation
Examples	Investigation of the chemical composition of a new insulin compound Survey of patients' views about women doctors	A randomised controlled trial of anything A retrospective comparison of one group exposed to a training programme compared to one group not receiving it	Developing a new home care service by the evaluator collaborating with providers to decide how to value the service and then collecting and feeding back data to them
Features	Focus: scientific knowledge Purpose: only to extend knowledge by filling gaps or resolving theoretical questions within the discipline by using scientific methods accepted by the discipline	Focus: scientific knowledge and practical decisions Purpose: helping practitioners (professionals and managers) to make decisions and contributing to scientific knowledge by using evaluation methods. Users are other scientists and practitioners	Focus: practical decisions. Purpose: enabling practitioners to make short-term decisions to improve their programme or reform. Less interest in generalisability of knowledge

planned and executed randomised controlled trials, are also scientific research. There is an overlap between evaluation and scientific research (*see* Table 1.1).

Systematic data gathering is another feature of the definition. This is common to both evaluation and pure scientific research, but in pure research the data to be collected are decided by the research questions, which in turn are decided by the gaps in knowledge or issues generated by theoretical debate within the discipline. In evaluation the data which are collected are the data which are important to the user. The user has certain criteria by which they judge the value of an intervention, such as cost or quick results.

This book uses the term 'data gathering' to describe many different ways to gather data, including measurement. Gathering people's perceptions about a programme or policy could be part of an evaluation and provide valid evidence, so long as this is done systematically and by following scientific methods which are accepted as capable of producing valid data.

Comparison is also an essential part of evaluations. We judge the value of something by making comparisons. Evaluations always involve comparisons of some type; either 'before' with 'after' or what was done with what was intended (e.g. with objectives or standards) or of one intervention with nothing or with a traditional intervention. For example, we may measure a patient's temperature but we cannot evaluate a patient's temperature unless we compare it with an average or with a previous measure of the same patient's temperature. We 'judge the value' of the patient's temperature by making a comparison. We do this to make a better informed decision, such as whether to give or stop giving antibiotics.

Box 1.4: Evaluation overlaps with other activities

- *Research* – systematic collection of data using scientific methods to discover new knowledge
- *Evaluation* – judging value by making a comparison (over time or between two or more things)
- *Measurement* – quantifying (you need two measures to evaluate something)
- *Monitoring* – continuous comparison of activity with a standard
- *Supervision* – for monitoring a person's work and training or for monitoring a health programme or policy
- *Quality assurance* – for identifying quality problems and resolving or preventing them

---

Table 1.2: Questions addressed by different types of evaluation

	Internal evaluation	*External independent evaluation*
Simple intervention	Has this patient benefited from my physiotherapy treatment?	Does this specific service meet the required standards?
Complex intervention	What are the outcomes of our integrated service for older people with health problems living at home?	What are the costs and outcomes of this health promotion programme?
		Has this reform been implemented and what are the results?

Types of evaluation

One reason why evaluation can be confusing is that there are so many types of evaluation such as formative, summative, process, impact, outcome, cost-utility, longitudinal case-control and audit evaluations. In 1987 Patton estimated that there were over 100 types of evaluation – there are probably more now! This book gives an introduction to the range of types by explaining the principles underlying the different approaches. It concentrates on process, outcome and action evaluations as these are the most useful for practising professionals, managers and policy makers. Here we note a few of the main types.

Programme feasibility assessment or option appraisal

These evaluations help to decide whether an action or programme should be carried out. Managers often request feasibility assessments to look at the possible benefits, risks and costs of a new service, a change to policy or a new technology. Those making the feasibility assessment may draw on evidence reported by evaluations carried out elsewhere of similar actions or interventions. Note that this is different from evaluation feasibility assessment discussed in Chapter 4, which is an assessment made by an evaluator as to whether it is feasible to do an evaluation.

Outcome evaluations or summative evaluation

Evaluations are often made of a programme or reform to discover its effects (outcome evaluations). Designs for doing this are described in Chapter 9. For some programmes the effects may not be obvious until some time in the future and therefore can be difficult to measure. The effects of health education on health take time to become apparent and it is usually difficult to be sure that the change in health status is due to the education and not to something else, such as higher income or better housing. The outcomes of health reforms are also difficult to measure. For these reasons evaluators sometimes make process evaluations.

Process evaluation or formative evaluation

Some evaluations consider how a programme or a reform was imple-mented, perhaps in order to discover what helped and hindered the implementation. This is because people may already know from previous evaluations that, if the change is implemented correctly, then certain results will follow. Another reason for undertaking a process evaluation is that outcomes may take some time to appear but we still want to find out if the programme is getting to the people for whom it was intended, whether it was implemented at all or whether it was implemented according to plans or regulations.

Designs for process evaluations are given in Chapter 8. Some quality evaluations or 'audits', which assess whether a service meets standards, are sometimes called process evaluations (*see* Chapter 13).

Action evaluation

Action evaluations are performed to give decision makers fast feedback about a programme or reform. The action evaluator works in close collaboration with the decision makers to help them define which information they need and then works closely with programme providers or change implementers to collect and check information about the programme and any effects as they occur. There is no attempt to control the programme or change process and the evaluator may give immediate feedback to those involved at different times to improve it.

What evaluation can and cannot do

- Evaluation itself cannot change anything, but it can give a more informed basis for others to make changes.
- An evaluation study cannot attribute value to the intervention, but it can give information which helps others to attribute value. In selecting which data to collect, the evaluator works with users to decide which information is relevant to judging the value of the thing they evaluate.
- Evaluation clarifies the criteria to be used to judge the value of the intervention.
- An evaluation study cannot include all the criteria which different people will use to judge the value of the intervention or all the things which people need to consider in deciding how to act.
- An evaluation does not have to be an expensive three-year randomised controlled trial; it can simply be a description of something such as a new policy and how it is implemented.

- Not all health evaluations look at effectiveness; there are other criteria of valuation such as whether standards were achieved.

Summary

- Evaluation is part of everyday healthcare. One aim of this book is to show practical ways to plan and carry out evaluations and to quickly make sense of an evaluation.
- Most attention has been given to evaluations of treatments and to medical research evaluation methods. Other activities and interventions such as programmes, policies and changes also need to be evaluated. There are many different methods which can be used to evaluate these, but which are not well understood in healthcare.
- We need to know if these 'non-treatment interventions' and changes make a difference for the people for whom they are intended, their impact on other people and the resources which they use. We also need to know something about how they are implemented and which factors help and hinder their success.
- This book describes an action research 'user-focused' approach which shows how evaluation can be linked to action, so that decisions, practice and health policies can be better informed. It shows how to concentrate on the evaluation user's informational needs and their value criteria, so as to make the evaluation more useful to them.
- An evaluation which cannot be used – such as to help make something more effective or less costly – is worse than useless because it takes time and money away from things that do make a difference.
- This book proposes that a single-user focused approach will produce more useful and conclusive results, although the users may want the evaluator to explore the perspectives of many stakeholders.
- Action evaluation is:
  - a service for a user/customer
  - to enable them to make more informed decisions
  - by systematically collecting data
  - which are relevant to the evaluation criteria which are important to them
  - and through making comparisons which enable value judgements.
- Evaluation is not measurement, but does use measures or data. Evaluation is a part of quality assurance and improvement.
- Some evaluation is research but not all research is evaluation.

Part 1

How to make an evaluation

Chapter 2

How to evaluate a health service or programme

Introduction

How would you evaluate a health service such as a primary healthcare centre? Or a programme such as health education for preventing heart disease?

There are six steps in carrying out an evaluation. In this chapter we look at the three most important: preparation, design planning and design choice. The other 'doing' steps are practical planning, data gathering and analysis, and reporting, described in Chapters 4 and 11.

There are many ways to make an evaluation, depending on how much time and resources you have and what the users of the evaluation want. The purpose of this chapter is to introduce evaluation tools by showing how to use them in a real example and to describe a standard approach which can be used for any service or programme evaluation. Later chapters will explain the tools in more detail but the aim here is to get started quickly and show a relatively simple way to carry out a user-focused evaluation.

After reading this chapter you will know which questions you need to answer to prepare for the evaluation and to plan the design. You will also see how to choose a design and get some ideas about data collection. A common mistake is to start gathering data without planning the evaluation. Many data are gathered without thinking about whether they will really help the users of the evaluation to make their decisions. This is why this chapter shows how to work through preparation, design planning and choice, before beginning to talk about methods for data collection.

The example is a rapid evaluation of an AIDS programme which I did with a colleague where a quarter of the population are HIV positive and will develop AIDS (Box 2.1). We could consider a simpler example, such as a primary care service for expectant mothers, but this example gives a good illustration of the trade-offs between the ideal way to evaluate a programme and what is feasible with the time and money available.

> **Box 2.1: How would you evaluate this programme? You have four weeks**
>
> Four projects were started in 1993 in different parts of an African country to care for people with AIDS and to prevent the transmission of HIV. The finance for these projects was provided by a Nordic donor aid agency to a churches association in the country. The churches association selected the four project sites, provided them with finance and supported the projects from a central unit. The four project sites were church hospitals, each of which set up project teams to provide the AIDS care and prevention services. Five evaluation team members were selected in 1999 to evaluate the four projects and the central support unit. The team had three months to prepare and then worked full time for four weeks on site to gather and analyse data.

Step 1: preparation

There are four questions to answer before you can decide the details of an evaluation.

- What are the constraints on the evaluation?
- Who are the stakeholders?
- Which criteria will be used to judge the value of the programme or service?
- What is the scope of the evaluation?

What are the constraints on the evaluation?

The three main constraints are:

- the timeframe (the length of time before the final report)
- the resources available for the evaluation, in terms of finance and people
- the data already collected by the programme which could be used in the evaluation.

In the AIDS evaluation, we had five full-time team members for one month of on-site work and three months before the on-site work for two team members to spend part time, planning the evaluation. There were few financial constraints on travel, but there were practical ones as three of the four sites were not easy to get to; travel would take up four days of the one month on site. The biggest constraint turned out to be the lack of documentation about what had been done at each site and about the incidence and prevalence of HIV/AIDS. More on this later when we consider the 'scope' of the evaluation.

There are always constraints on an evaluation which limit what can be done (the 'scope' of the evaluation); for example, how many different types of data sources can be used and what levels of detail and accuracy are possible. By clarifying these at the outset, you can be realistic about what can be done. You might even decide not to proceed because you will not learn enough from the evaluation to give valid or useful information to its users.

Who are the stakeholders?

The 'stakeholders' are people and groups with an interest in the programme or service or people who are affected by it in some way. In the example, there were people with AIDS or who were HIV positive, employees of the project, the funding agency, the churches association which was managing the projects and the hospitals which 'hosted' each project. There can be many stakeholders, not just those who are aware of their interest in the programme: many villagers and other groups were not aware that they had 'a stake' in it.

Why the need to list the stakeholders when preparing for the evaluation? First, to decide which stakeholders are the 'primary users' of the evaluation. These are the people for whom the evaluation is intended and who need the evaluation to make better informed decisions. The evaluation should ideally be designed for one user group with their decisions in mind. Trying to meet the needs of all users will not meet anyone's needs and result in gathering too much data and a poor and confused evaluation. It is difficult enough to decide a design to meet the needs of one user group.

Note that the evaluation user may not be the patients or other users of the programme or service user. In the example, the evaluation users were the funding agency, the churches association and each project team. The programme or service users were people with AIDS or HIV positive, their families and carers and the general population.

Which criteria will be used to judge the value of the programme or service?

The evaluation value criteria are what the users of the evaluation think is important to know about the programme. In the example, the primary user was the funding agency. They used the 'six criteria' method to judge the value of the programme.

1 Whether the actual programme was implemented as planned in the proposal (compliance).
2 The extent to which it met its objectives (achievement of objectives).
3 The results of the programme for people with AIDS, those who were HIV positive and the general population (target outcomes).
4 How relevant and appropriate the activities were to people's needs (relevance).
5 How many resources were used and whether they were used properly (efficiency).
6 Whether the programme was sustainable (sustainability).

To find out how the programme performed on these criteria, each criterion needs to be further specified so as to decide which data to collect. This is done in the later evaluation planning stage. The first thing, though, is to list these main value criteria. This means the evaluator has to talk to the evaluation user to agree the important criteria for judging the value of the programme or service. They rarely have these explicitly formulated and often need help to define what is important to them and why they need to know this. Showing them the six criteria above can help users to decide what they most need to know. Later chapters discuss how to help evaluation users to define their criteria and whether you can include other criteria such as those of other stakeholders. Users and stakeholders always want many more criteria to be investigated than are possible given the time and money for the evaluation.

What is the scope of the evaluation?

The scope of the evaluation defines what will and will not be studied. For example, whether to use a 'wide-angle lens' to look at the programme and its results in general or whether to use a 'telephoto lens' to look at parts in more detail. You cannot do both because of limited time and money.

First, the main outlines of the 'thing' to be evaluated have to be decided. In the example, this was what people carrying out the programme had been doing – the programme component 'activities'. The evaluator needs to be clear about what the programme is and what it is not. In the example, we were not sure at first if one AIDS training programme for school teachers was part of the programme to be evaluated. Another question is the period over which the programme is to be studied: often it is from the start of the programme to the time the evaluation is started, which in the example was six years.

The second aspect of the scope of the evaluation is to decide the 'breadth' of the outcomes to be studied. The breadth is the timescale over which the outcomes are studied and the coverage, as well as how many different outcomes will be studied. The timescale covers whether to look at the immediate results of the programme, such as how many people were treated or trained, or whether to look at longer term results such as changes in knowledge or behaviour or even in health status.

The user's evaluation criteria show the ideal scope of the evaluation. For example, in the AIDS evaluation one criterion was whether objectives were met and one set of objectives was for the programme to train personnel on how to protect themselves from HIV infection. If this were the only way the users judged the programme then the scope of the evaluation would be narrow. But other criteria made the scope very wide: what were the results of the programme for different people? This means looking at short- and long-term outcomes for people with AIDS, people who were HIV positive and for the population.

Our mistake was not to limit the scope further because in practice it proved difficult properly to collect reliable data about all the criteria at all the sites in the time available, in part because the projects did not have the data already collected and documented. This takes us to one of the important ways to define the scope of the evaluation: find out which data have already been collected and are available for the evaluation. If there are no or few data collected by the programme, then the scope of the evaluation will have to be more limited: the evaluator will have to try to gather data first hand, rather than using programme documentation or statistics, and this takes time.

Thus a key question to help decide the scope is: 'Can the evaluator use previously collected data and existing information systems, or is it likely that they will have to gather primary data?' The evaluator needs to clarify which data and documentation are available about the programme. This included a written plan and data about the inputs to the programme (e.g. how many personnel?), its processes or activities (are these documented in records or in procedures?) and its outputs (e.g. how many patients treated?) and outcomes (e.g. records of the results of treatment). In our example, we knew from previous experience that project records would not be detailed and that data about the number of people with AIDS or HIV positive would be unreliable. In the early stages we asked questions about documentation and did not get clear answers, so we assumed that we would have to look hard for documentation at each site and that we might not find any. Finding out which data are already available can be done through questioning key people and involves assessing the accessibility, validity and reliability of these data.

As always, there is the 'evaluation compromise': the balance between the ideal and the feasible. One of the reasons for working through these preparation questions is for the evaluator to consider what is possible and then to help the user of the evaluation to clarify exactly what they want from the evaluation and what they can expect from it. These four preparation questions help to determine what type of evaluation is needed and what is possible. Detailed answers are not necessary early on, just notes and ideas to start the thinking and planning process. The questions help to identify what you need to find out more about in order properly to plan the evaluation.

Step 2: design planning

The next step is to decide the design of the evaluation. To do this the evaluation needs to answer six questions about the programme or service.

1 What are the 'boundaries and components' of the programme to be evaluated?

This question makes us define the 'thing' to be evaluated in a more precise way than when we asked the initial questions about scope. We had already excluded the teacher's education programme, so some of the boundaries had been drawn. The boundaries are where we draw the line between the activities of the programme we are evaluating and other activities which we will not include as part of the programme.

The next part is deciding the components of the programme. There were four projects, each located at a different place, as well as the activities of the central unit to support the projects. Were there therefore five component parts? We could have said 'yes', but we decided that each project had similar component parts which we would have to study at each site. Before visiting, we read the programme's statement of objectives and interviewed personnel at the central support unit. We found that each project had the same range of activities, which are listed

Table 2.1: Data checklist

Programme components	Data about inputs and activities	Data about results
Home care service		
Counselling service		
AIDS/HIV health education services		
Assistance to orphans		
Traditional midwives and healers support		
Schools services		
Blood testing, equipment and supplies		
Management		

in Table 2.1. Once we had defined the components we made a data-gathering checklist to remind us that we had to gather data about each component to describe it and the results.

2 Who is the 'target' of the programme?

This question asks the evaluator to define who the programme is for or who it is supposed to benefit. The targets of the AIDS programme were the people living in the project areas, and specifically people with AIDS, people who were HIV positive and their carers, high-risk populations, as well as the general population. The targets of the central support unit were the project personnel at each site, who were in need of training, support and supplies as well as finance. We could see from this preparatory question that there would be issues about priorities: how many resources are allocated to the activities for different target groups?

It is useful if you can define the primary intended targets – the main people for whom the programme is intended. This is not always possible as few programmes set priorities between different groups. Often the evaluator discovers who in practice are the priority targets and can point this out to the evaluation user so that they can decide if this really should be the priority target group.

3 What are the intended 'target outcomes'?

What difference did the programme make for the targets? This question asks the evaluator to define in what way the target is supposed to be different as a result of the programme. For example, patients should have reduced symptoms or a complete cure. The outcomes for the targets may be stated in the original programme proposal or there may be objectives which give some clues about the intended outcomes for the targets. The 1993 AIDS programme proposal had some statements, but they described objectives at different levels of abstraction and also included statements about programme activities.

> *5.1 Development objectives: prevention of HIV infection.*
>
> *5.2 Intermediate objectives: number of HIV-positive persons reduced, number of home-based care patients increased, number of AIDS patients occupying hospital beds reduced.*
>
> *5.3 Intermediate objectives: number of HIV-positive persons stabilised, spread of HIV infection from urban and mining areas to the countryside reduced, HIV-infected blood trans-fusions avoided, home-based care improved, costs of care reduced.*
>
> *5.4 Programme support objectives: home-based care improved, counselling improved, training improved.*

Using these statements, we defined the main target outcomes as being to prevent or reduce the spread of HIV in the population and to provide care and counselling to people with HIV or AIDS.

Programmes have many outcomes, some intended and some not, some outcomes for targets and some outcomes for other people such as health personnel – these are all the 'results' of the programme. No evaluation has the time or resources to gather data about all outcomes. One way to limit the evaluation to what is feasible is to gather data about intended outcomes for the targets: most evaluation users are interested in the difference the programme makes for the people it is intended to serve.

Note that there were other statements about objectives in the pro-gramme proposal. Because one of the criteria was how well objectives were met, we recognised that we would need to gather evidence to check if all of these objectives had been met.

4   Which 'target outcome data' could we collect?

Another way of putting this question is: 'Which data could we collect to find out if the programme made a difference for the targets, given the time and resources we have?' The programme could have had many different effects on just one target group, for example the people with AIDS. If we also consider the outcomes for other targets – health personnel, the local population, carers of people with AIDS – we can see that we would need to collect a large amount of data. This question thus asks the evaluator to decide which specific outcomes to consider and how to collect data about these outcomes. There are four ways to decide which data to collect.

- Focus first on the primary targets of the programme (e.g. people with AIDS).
- Decide which outcomes are of interest to the users of the evaluation (e.g. AIDS patients' satisfaction with the programme).
- Decide which data are available and how much time it will take to collect and analyse them (e.g. no available data, so we need time to interview a sample of AIDS patients).
- Decide how to assess whether the outcomes really are the result of the programme and not something else (e.g. will AIDS patients know if it was the AIDS programme which helped them or some other service?). Another way to put this is: do not waste time collecting data about outcomes which you cannot prove were caused by the programme.

Finding data about outcomes proved to be the biggest difficulty in the AIDS evaluation. The national studies giving data about the incidence of HIV and AIDS were dubious. They showed HIV rates of between 9% and 27% in populations of expectant mothers and the methods for measurement had changed over the years. These data could not be extrapolated to the populations at the four very different sites and there were no data about HIV or AIDS incidence or prevalence collected at these sites.

Was lack of data a failure of the AIDS projects? Should they have regularly collected data about incidence through surveys? This requirement was not in the statement of objectives for the programme and it was generally thought that money was better spent on other things. In effect, there were no 'before' and 'after' data which is one thing an evaluator looks for when planning design; for example, about the number of HIV-positive people in the project areas. Even if there were, it would have been difficult in the time to assess whether the projects or other factors had caused a before–after change.

We decided that the data we would have to use were judgements made by different informants about:

- whether HIV and AIDS would be more widespread without the programmes and by how much
- whether the people most needing care and counselling were getting it
- what would have happened without the programme.

We used the technique of asking informants why they took the view they did and if they knew of any evidence which would contradict or support their judgements because it was our task to report this evidence.

Africans who could not read and write readily understood the concept of independent evidence, when asked in the right way by my African evaluator colleagues.

5 What are the 'unintended outcomes'? (How can we discover other important outcomes?)

This question asks: 'How can we find out if the intervention has made some things worse or has indirect benefits?' The earlier questions forced the evaluator to be realistic about how much and which data they could collect and to concentrate on a few outcomes for the targets. This question also works in the opposite direction to ask how the evaluator can capture other 'important' outcomes which were not expected. Another way to use this is to think of the evaluator 'fishing' for data: which data and sources is it feasible to use in 'spreading our net' to catch a wide enough range of outcomes?

The method we used in the AIDS evaluation was to ask informants for their assessment of both the positive and negative results of the programme. The quality of the evaluation data about outcomes depended on us interviewing a wide range of different informants. In our preparations, we tried to arrange interviews with different representatives, both individually and in groups, and without the project personnel being present.

6 What are the 'confounders' or alternative explanations for the outcomes? (How do we know that something else did not cause the outcomes?)

Anyone reading the evaluation report will be thinking of all the other things which could explain any outcomes which the evaluator discovers. This last 'design-planning' question asks the evaluator to consider and try to exclude other explanations for any outcomes which they may discover. All evaluations have to wrestle with this 'problem of attribution'.

In our evaluation, changes in the incidence and prevalence of HIV and AIDS in the target populations could be caused by many things apart from the programme. In our preparation for the AIDS evaluation we studied the history of the project from reports and considered the changes taking place in the healthcare and economy of the country for the years before and during the projects. We listed other likely explanations for the outcomes such as health programmes run by others, national government campaigns, economic changes affecting migration and travel and changes to local customs such as traditional healing practices which can transmit HIV. We could not exclude any of these explanations, but we knew that in our report we had to try to assess their likely impact. The main data we used to assess these factors came from local and national informants in response to questions asking them to assess the impact of these factors.

You can never prove for certain that an outcome was caused by the programme and not by something else, even if you use an evaluation design which controls for all the factors you could imagine as having an influence. This 'problem of attribution' is one of the main challenges for a programme evaluation: how to assess the impact of other factors which may have caused any change to the target which the evaluator may have been able to document. This issue takes us to the subject of evaluation design, the third step in planning an evaluation.

Step 3: design choice

Answering the design-planning questions above gives the basis for deciding which type of evaluation design to use. The choice is between four types of design which are discussed in more detail in later chapters (*see* Box 2). Which of these do you think we used in the AIDS evaluation?

Box 2.2: Designs for evaluating health programmes

- Describe what was done and the strengths and weaknesses of the programme activities (type 1)
- Compare programme activities in relation to objectives and standards (type 2)
- Compare before with after (type 3)
- Compare one site with other(s) (type 4)

Type 1: descriptive

This design aims to gather data to describe the programme activities and how they may have changed over the years. It does not attempt to measure outcomes, but will note informants' views about positive and negative consequences and what helped and hindered the programme implementation. This design is useful for documenting the history of a programme or where the boundaries or components of the programme or service are not clear.

One framework to guide data gathering is to describe inputs and structure (e.g. number and type of personnel, how they are organised), processes/activities (e.g. providing direct care, education talks) and outputs in quantitative and qualitative terms (e.g. 120 patients treated a month). This design is also useful where sponsors of an evaluation are not clear exactly what they want evaluated. It can help to define what is and what is not the programme or policy, which can then be studied using other designs (e.g. a descriptive study can be phase 1 of a longer evaluation). The AIDS example used this design in part because the exact details of what was being done in the programme had not been clearly described. However, the evaluation users also wanted to know if objectives and standards had been met, which required the type 2 audit design.

Type 2: audit

This design compares what is being done (the 'activities') with what was planned, with objectives or standards or with a model. There are four types of audit design.

Audit type A: audit against plan and objective

This design takes the programme proposal with its statement of objectives and the 'measurables', where these are specified (e.g. all AIDS patients will be visited every week) and investigates the extent to which these plans have been carried out and explains the findings (e.g. why some things were not carried out and why some planned activities were 'successful' while some 'failed'). In the AIDS evaluation we took the many objectives stated in the proposal and assessed whether the programme had achieved these. A common problem is where there is no a programme proposal document or the objectives are not well stated; they may need to be inferred by the evaluator and checked with managers.

Audit type B: audit against specified standards

This is a 'process evaluation' design which describes the programme and compares what was done with specific standards or procedures. In the AIDS evaluation we had to check whether financial and other regulations for distributing and accounting for supplies had been met.

Audit type C: audit against a model

As with the other types of audit, this type first describes what was done but then compares this against an 'expert's' model for the programme or activity. For example, the evaluator takes an expert's model of an ideal training programme and then compares this with what people did in the programme. This design was used in an evaluation of the Norwegian total quality management programme; a model of total quality management which was described in the literature was used and the hospital quality programmes were compared to this model (Øvretveit, 1999).

Audit type D: audit against the evaluator's model of what was intended

The evaluator takes broad plans and intentions from documents and interviews, creates a model of the programme or policy and its expected outcomes (possibly validating this with clients at an early stage) and then compares what happened with this model.

None of these audit designs questions whether the programme is the right one. They just compare what happens with plans, specifications or models: they are 'compliance evaluations'. A programme may be carried out as intended but may have negative consequences or not meet people's needs and this might not be discovered with this design. Audit designs ask 'Did they do things right?' (as specified), not 'Did they do the right things?' (meeting needs with the fewest resources). Type 3 designs look at needs before and after the intervention.

Type 3: before and after (outcome) – simple

This design aims to gather data about the target before and after the intervention (or before and 'later' if the intervention continues). The target can be one population group at 'time 1' and the same group some time later at 'time 2' or it can be one group of patients at 'time 1' and another group who received the same programme at a later 'time 2'. The target of the intervention is usually patients or citizens but it can be health personnel (e.g. design 6a in Chapter 9) or even all three, as in the AIDS evaluation.

In rapid evaluations, both the 'before' (baseline) and 'after' data are collected from statistics and retrospectively after the intervention has been carried out. This depends on data-gathering systems being in place or on an informant's memory of 'before' and 'after' states (which can be more reliable than some data-gathering systems). In order not to mislead the users of the evaluation, studies of this type must investigate and clearly state the limitations of the data sources (validity and reliability) and also list the other possible causes of any 'before–after' differences, apart from the intervention which was evaluated (the 'attribution' challenge noted earlier).

It is costly and difficult to gather data about the needs of targets before and after. Therefore these designs often have to concentrate on limited indicators of need, such as how many people used a service out of an estimate of how many needed it.

Ideally, the data needed to assess the impact of the intervention should be decided and gathered before a programme is started. Managers implementing the programme need training on which data they will need to monitor the programme and how to set up systems to do this. In practice, those overseeing the programme at higher levels may need to specify the data required and even the design of the data system and make funding dependent on recipients showing that the data-gathering systems are in place and will be functioning to monitor the project. Funders should consider building capacity to both implement and monitor the programme, rather than arranging for external evaluations with separate data-gathering exercises.

Type 4: comparative (outcome)

This design gathers data about the target before and after the programme, like the type 3 design. But in addition it compares this to data about targets receiving another type of programme (or nothing) at a 'control site'. For example, we can gather data about people before and after receiving a health programme in one place and compare this with similar people who did not receive a health programme in another place. In effect, this design is a 'double' type 3. It is more expensive because we have to collect and analyse twice the data about outcomes. We also have to check how similar the two groups of people are so that we can assess explanations for different outcomes being due to the type of people served rather than the different programmes. Ideally we should try to ensure that the people at both sites are similar through 'matching'.

Summary: how to carry out a service or programme evaluation

This chapter described three steps for planning an evaluation: preparation, design planning and design choice. Once this planning work is done then the three practical steps follow: practical planning (step 4), data gathering and analysis (step 5), and reporting (step 6). More detail on these steps are given in Chapters 4, 11 and 12. The summary below shows how these steps were followed in the example under the three headings of programme definition, deciding evaluation criteria and collecting data.

Programme definition

The first question is: 'What is the service or programme and its objectives?' In the AIDS evaluation we asked: 'Is the programme actually a number of projects at one place or at different sites?' And what are the component parts of the programme?

We defined the programme as the services of the central support unit to the four projects and the activities of the four projects, such as direct home care to people with AIDS and school services. We created this definition by using the descriptions in the programme documents and by talking to the central unit personnel. To define the intended objectives, we used what was written in the programme proposal. This listed many different aims. Some were abstract, such as reducing the number of deaths from AIDS, and some specific, such as training all personnel on how to protect themselves from infection. Some were activities, such as supplying condoms, some were outcomes in measurable terms, such as all patients with AIDS should receive a visit every week. We used a model for structuring objectives which separates higher order objectives from lower order ones, activities from outcomes and short-term from long-term outcomes (Appendix 6).

In our report we described what we had defined as the objectives and explained what we had done to assess progress in achieving these objectives (we asked stakeholders what they thought the objectives were and how far they thought these had been achieved and what evidence they had for saying this). We suggested how to make objectives clearer in the future.

If you are carrying out an evaluation, your first question is: 'What are we to evaluate and what are its objectives?' Decide which activities you will not be evaluating (which are outside the boundary of the service or programme), what are the components and what you will take the objectives to be. Finish your definition of the programme by noting any synergy – how the different activities of the programme interact to support each other, or which duplicate or undermine each other. Consider how to assess activities which overlap components, such as management, supervision and training; will you make them separate components or part of each component?

Deciding evaluation criteria

Next, decide which criteria you will use to judge the value of the programme. We used a standard six criteria which can be used to evaluate any health service or programme. If the evaluation users are not sure how they want to judge the value of the programme, these six give a basis for helping to clarify what is important for users to know about a programme.

1 *Description of the programme* and divergence from programme proposal or plan.
2 *Achievement of objectives* – to what extent were objectives achieved?
3 *Outcomes* – what difference did the programme make to the target people and different stakeholders? Coverage?
4 *Relevance and appropriateness* – were the activities relevant to changing needs and technically and culturally appropriate?
5 *Efficiency* – how many resources were put in (time and money), was there any avoidable waste, could more outputs have been achieved with the resource inputs, would a small extra amount of resources have produced disproportionately larger benefits (marginal input benefits), what were the opportunity costs?
6 *Sustainability* – with and without continued finance. What are the risks and what are the strengths?

Agreeing evaluation criteria also involves saying what is feasible. In the example, we tried to gather data for all these six criteria at each project. Given our time and resources and the data available, this meant we could only gather a little data about each one; we went for coverage to give a general picture, rather than depth and validity. One of the four preparation questions is about how much time and resources you have. The more information the users want, the more the evaluation will cost and the longer it will take, so when discussing evaluation criteria, there is a trade-off between the number of criteria and the cost and time of the evaluation.

Data collection

Planning data collection means deciding which data you need to give evidence about the performance of the programme against the criteria. In the example, we collected data from different sources: project management documents and from different people. We needed to think about how we would get access to these sources and which sample of people we would ideally like to interview. Before going on the field visit we had a plan of who we wanted to see, a checklist data collection form and also a semi-structured questionnaire based on the six criteria (Appendix 5).

Thinking about evidence is not just thinking about data sources and methods for collecting and analysing data. Evidence means evidence about the programme or service and not about something else. How can we be more certain that the apparent outcomes of the programme are actually due to the programme and not something else?

So, when planning data collection, use the value criteria to decide which data you need, look at your design choices and the time, money and user's questions you need to answer and decide a design which is feasible and answers as many as possible of these questions.

Data collection for the 'six criteria' method

We finish this chapter by giving a guide for using the standard six criteria method for evaluating any service or programme which focuses on which data to collect. First the method asks how you plan to collect data to describe the intervention.

Description of the service or programme?

Which data do you need in order to describe the service or programme as it was actually carried out as well as any changes which may have happened to it over the period which your evaluation has to consider? From which sources will you collect these data and which methods will you use to collect the data to describe the programme? This description has to be accurate enough for the reader to understand key details of the service or programme, how it is similar and different from other programmes and, ideally, to be able to replicate the programme if they chose to.

Correspondence to objectives and procedures?

This question asks which data you need to assess whether the programme in practice corresponded to the objectives or standards set for it or to any procedures laid down for how it should be carried out (e.g. were financial accounting procedures met?). By asking this question the evaluator can plan which data sources to go to and how to collect, record and analyse these data to assess whether the programme met this criterion of correspondence.

Outcomes?

This question asks which data are needed to find out what difference the programme made to both the target people and to other key people. The evaluation plan can show which types of data will be collected about short-term and long-term outcomes and whether any 'before data' will be collected (data about targets before the programme).

	Short-term outcomes	*Long-term outcomes*
Objective data (e.g. before and after measures)		
Subjective data (e.g. informant's perception retrospectively)		

Efficiency?

Most evaluation users want the evaluator to collect data about the resources consumed by the programme and the number of outputs produced; for example, the cost per person treated or educated. This question directs the evaluator's attention to how they can find out how much time and money were consumed by the programme and how outputs can be measured. It is also useful to compare this 'cost–output efficiency ratio' to that of an alternative, including nothing. This draws the user's attention to what they sacrificed by using their resources for this programme rather than another – the 'opportunity cost' of the programme.

Acceptability?

This question directs attention to which data could be collected to assess people's willingness to use the service or programme, in the short and long-term. Also, which data do you need to assess the technical and cultural acceptability of the programme to the people who have to implement it and carry out the activities?

Sustainability?

This question covers the plan to collect data about three aspects of the 'sustainability' of the programme. The first is which factors threaten the continuation of the programme, if finance continues. The second is whether the programme could be continued if special financing were withdrawn. A third question is how to get data about what helped to sustain the start of the programme; what were the conditions and factors necessary to start the programme and which factors greatly assisted the start?

An additional question could be added to look at management performance as a separate item. The long-term results of good performance are that the most important needs are met and no resources are wasted. However, it is often difficult to assess this (although you can assess if there was waste). We usually assess the management processes which are thought to result in good performance, usually including whether management followed the programme planning and operation requirements. Areas to consider are clarity and appropriateness of programme structure (vertical and lateral co-ordination), quality of planning and budgeting, adequacy of systematic reviews of resource management and replanning (involving cost–benefit assessment of different sub-programmes), adequacy of documentation, monitoring and reporting, accuracy and standards of financial accounting, performance in supplies management and personnel management, and compliance with higher level programme management requirements.

Appendix 5 gives guidance questions for gathering data about the performance of the programme against each of these criteria.

Box 2.3: Summary of the 'six criteria' method for evaluating a health programme

- What did they do (description) and how did this diverge from the proposal and plan?
- Did they achieve the objectives (correspondence to objectives)?
- Did they meet people's needs (outcomes)?
- Did they waste any resources or could they have used resources more efficiently (efficiency)?
- Did people use the service (acceptability)?
- What threatens the continuation – with and without continued funding (sustainability)?

Summary

- This chapter gave guidance on how to carry out an evaluation of a service or programme and introduced evaluation tools through an example. Later chapters explain the concepts and designs in more detail.
- Design the evaluation for one group of evaluation users by finding out how they value the intervention and what they need to know to make decisions.
- Time, money and available data limit what an evaluation can do: preparation means clarifying these constraints and discussing with users what is feasible and what they most need from the evaluation.
- The first three steps of an evaluation are: preparation, design planning and deciding design.
- **Step 1.** Preparation involves deciding the constraints to the evaluation, the stakeholders, which criteria will be used to judge the value of the programme or service and the scope of the evaluation.
- **Step 2.** Design planning involves answering six questions:
  1 What are the 'boundaries and components' of the item or action to be evaluated?
  2 What is the 'target' of the programme or action to be evaluated?
  3 What are the 'target outcomes' or the difference the programme is expected to make to the target?
  4 Which 'target outcome data' could we collect? How can we know if the intervention has made a difference to the target?
  5 How can we discover other important outcomes?
  6 What are the alternative explanations for the outcomes? How do we know that something else did not cause the outcomes?
- **Step 3.** Deciding design involves choosing between four types of design: descriptive (where it is not clear exactly what the programme is), audit (where the programme intentions are described and evaluation users want to know if these intentions were met), before and after (to find out what the outcomes might be), comparative before and after (to compare outcomes with other programmes or with nothing).
- One way to evaluate a programme is to assess it against the six criteria of: 1 description of the programme and correspondence to what was proposed or planned; 2 achievement of objectives; 3 outcomes; 4 relevance and appropriateness; 5 efficiency; and 6 sustainability.
- The last three steps of an evaluation are practical planning, data gathering and analysis and reporting. These are considered in Chapters 4, 11 and 12.

Chapter 3

How to evaluate a policy, change or reform to healthcare

It is striking how little is known about the effectiveness and cost effectiveness of interventions that change the practice or delivery of healthcare. (Bero *et al.*, 1998)

Reforms and policies cannot be evaluated – only the implementation plan and actions can be evaluated.

Introduction

Healthcare changes or reforms are different from health programmes because they aim to change how healthcare organisations work, rather than intervening directly with patients or populations. An example of a change to organisation is computerising a patient records system. Examples of reforms are the many decentralisation reforms carried out in the Nordic countries (Alban and Christiansen, 1995; Brogren and Brommels, 1990; Hakkinen, 1997).

Reform is another word for change but we usually think of a reform as a large-scale change of national or regional scope. Reforms may also be small scale and local, such as two hospitals merging to reform hospital care in one area. Some policies are changes and also reforms, such as a new policy about giving patients more information about treatments. This policy aims to change how personnel behave and healthcare organisations operate. The point is that there is a category of things which aim to change healthcare organisation and which need to be evaluated. This category includes small changes, reforms and many policies.

Healthcare reforms are different from health reforms because they aim to change healthcare rather than to improve health. However, some healthcare reforms aim to do both. A reform to promote the use of quality methods in a healthcare organisation may aim to both reduce costs and improve clinical outcomes, which improves health. Some 'purchasing reforms' aim ultimately to benefit patients (Anell & Svarvar, 1993; Bergman, 1998; Saltman *et al.*, 1998). Many changes and reforms to healthcare have better patient care as one outcome but in some cases the aim may be to save money.

This chapter gives six steps of guidance for evaluating a healthcare change or reform: define the change, evaluation perspective, design, gather data, consider explanations and report. After reading this chapter you will be able to follow these six steps to plan an evaluation of a change or a reform. You will also know how to deal with the two challenges of:

- describing exactly what the change or reform was
- discovering effects which can unambiguously be attributed to the change or reform.

Part of the problem is deciding what is the reform and what is the implementation and whether both will be considered as the reform 'intervention'. Often reforms and policies do not give a detailed implementation plan: people have to interpret and plan local implementation actions. Another challenge is deciding what is the reform and what are the effects. This chapter includes models which help separate the reform 'instrument' from the reform implementation and short-term from long-term effects so as to describe the way a reform is carried out (Boxes 3.3 and 3.5).

Box 3.1: What is a healthcare reform?

A significant change introduced by national or local government legislation to the financing, organisation or functioning of health care services or to patients rights. (Øvretveit, 1998b)

A purposive dynamic and sustained process that results in systematic structural change. (WHO, 1996)

Saltman and Figueras (1997) categorise reform strategies as addressing: 1 resource scarcity (containing aggregate spending); 2 third-party payer issues (financing collection and operation); 3 provider payment and allocation of finance; 4 provider services (efficiency/quality).

Why evaluate changes or reforms?

The reasons for evaluating a proposed change or reform before it is started are to assess whether it is feasibile, to predict problems and to help plan how to implement it. This is 'formative evaluation' and can be done by piloting the change in one area or by making a 'paper evaluation' which draws on evidence from evaluations of similar changes elsewhere. During a change the reason for making an evaluation is to allow corrections during the implementation. After a change (or later in the process of change), an evaluation helps to discover the lessons for future changes or reforms and to contribute to scientific knowledge. A more immediate reason is to hold politicians and managers to account for changes which they made or did not make.

Evaluating a reform usually involves:

- describing the reform 'instrument' (e.g. a law, which states intentions) and implementation process (what was actually done) or the policy document
- gathering data about changes in health service performance and possibly also in health (outcome data)
- assessing whether these data really are outcomes of the reform (i.e. assessing the extent to which the reform or policy caused or influenced the changes registered in the outcome indicators).

The aim is often to:

- present evidence of the results of the reform or policy
- describe the process of implementing the reform or policy
- assess the strengths and weaknesses of the reform or policy as implemented and judge the value of the results (in relation to the criteria of valuation used in the evaluation)
- recommend improvements.

Reform is an intentional change to organisation

The mental health decentralisation reform in Norway was an 'intentional change' to the responsibilities of counties and of the smaller communes within the counties. A law transferred responsibilities for general care for people with mental health problems from the counties 'downwards' to communes. Like other reforms, it was an 'intervention' which was planned and had a managed implementation process, although there were different views about how well this was done.

In most reforms the intention is to change organisation, procedures, financing methods and other factors. These are termed the 'immediate target' of the reform intervention – the thing which the intervention acts on directly and aims to change in the short term. But there is often an aim beyond changing health organisations or financing methods; the long-term aim is often to make services better for patients (e.g. more accessible and responsive) or to improve patients' health or well-being, which are more difficult to assess. In the following, these 'ultimate beneficiaries' are termed the 'ultimate target' of the change.

Not all healthcare reforms have this aim. For those that do, the intervention does not work directly on the ultimate targets (patients or the population) but works through changing the immediate target (health organisation) in order to achieve the ultimate benefits of better health. (This is shown in Figure 9.5.)

The purposes of such intentional changes are usually to save money, improve quality, increase production, efficiency or effectiveness. There are often multiple purposes, such as to reduce public expenditure, increase efficiency and choice and make services more responsive to patients. The complexity of health reforms is a challenge to the evaluator as they need to describe exactly the reform that was implemented, not what the reform was on paper. The following gives an example of the difficulty of defining a reform.

> *We are introducing a change to our procedures, which is intended to change how our personnel act, in order to change how patients take care of themselves. The aim is to improve the health of the population. We do not expect other significant changes to occur, but some may be unavoidable.*

Which of the changes is the intervention we should evaluate, and which are changes to the target? Which other changes might the evaluators study? The statement has the advantage of describing different components and some components may be viewed as part of the reform to be evaluated. It can be used to map a reform sequence or causal chain model; these are methods which evaluators use to define a reform. We can separate the different changes which were made (components) and also draw a causal chain model of events over time and their interaction. The next section starts with a simple model to help separate the intervention from the target (Box 3.3), and drawing the EITO diagram is also a good first step (*see* Box 6.3). Box 3.2 gives five questions for separating the different things to be studied.

Box 3.2: How to describe a health reform, change or policy

To explain a health reform describe:

- *what* was changed (the 'target' of the reform – the thing the reform directly worked upon, which is different from the intended ultimate outcome) (e.g. hospital financing method)
- *the target before and after* (from what to what?)
- *how* (what was the intervention which was made?)
- *why* (what was the purpose, objective and end result intended (intermediate and ultimate outcome)?)
- *how* could we know if the reform was successful? (data, value criteria)

Illustration: a decentralisation reform changed the responsibilities of Swedish counties and communes (the target), so that communes took over from the counties responsibilities for the care of older people (the targets before and after). The reform was carried out by legislation and a detailed implementation programme (how the intervention was made), for the purposes of providing care more locally and efficiently (the outcomes). Indicators of success and failure are change in costs, complaints and satisfaction of patient groups and providers' assessment of the process and the outcome.

Step 1: define the change

The rest of this chapter gives six steps to follow to evaluate a health reform. The people introducing the change – the 'reformers' – might not define the subjects discussed in each step, but these subjects need to be clearly defined by the evaluator. The general model which helps to define the change is shown in Box 3.3.

Box 3.3: A simple causal chain model of a reform

Reform intervention (e.g. a new law or a reform implementation process) $\Rightarrow$ Immediate target of reform (e.g. health personnel) $\Rightarrow$ Ultimate target (e.g. citizens, patients, population) $\Rightarrow$ Collect data about *effect* on immediate target (e.g. did personnel change their behaviour?) and *impact* on ultimate target (e.g. what was the effect on patients?)

In the first step the evaluator needs to define the reform intervention, the targets and the characteristics of the targets to be examined. The questions in Box 3.2 and the model in Box 3.3 help the evaluator to separate and define these different subjects.

The reform intervention is what specifically was changed and how it was changed. A reform, change or policy cannot itself be evaluated. Only the real actions which real people take in response can be evaluated: the implementation plans and actions. In one sense this is an extreme statement because in a general way one can evaluate a general reform, change or policy statement. However, it makes the point that it is the specific implementation actions which should be evaluated. And, of course, there may be questions about how well the plan interpreted the general reform or policy statement. Take an example of a reform to decentralise non-specialist care for people with mental health problems from a region (e.g. a county) to a community (e.g. a commune). The intervention is both the law (the reform 'instrument') and the different actions people took to transfer services, personnel and finance from counties to communes (the implementation actions). Each local area prepares their own plan. Then they implement it. Thus one could evaluate (i) the reform, change or policy instrument, (ii) the plan for implementation, (iii) the steps taken in reality (which may be none at all). The emphasis of most evaluations is on the latter.

Another question is were the planning and preparations made before the law was implemented also part of the intervention? Were the discussions between counties and communes about what might change also part of the intervention, even before it was clear that the law would be proposed? These are questions which the evaluator and others must answer in order to draw the boundaries around the intervention to be evaluated.

The 'immediate target' is, who or what should be different as a direct and immediate result of this intervention. For example, a procedure for allocating finance should be changed or part of an organisation is changed or health personnel are to behave differently. In the example the immediate targets are personnel and county and commune organisation and financing. The 'ultimate target' of the change is the group of people who should ultimately benefit from the change (e.g. patients or populations). In the example this is people with mental health problems or those at risk of such problems.

One last question needs to be answered to define the reform changes. What is the intended immediate effect of the reform on the target? This asks exactly how the immediate target is supposed to be different as a result of the intervention. If the decentralisation was done successfully, what would people do differently or how would the procedure or organisation structure be different after, compared with before the intervention?

The 'intended impact on the ultimate target' is the difference which the intervention intends to make for patients or populations. Often the 'objectives' of the intervention are defined in terms of the intended impact on the ultimate or immediate targets; for example, patients get the care they need more quickly or local personnel have more decision-making authority.

Box 3.4: Summary of step 1 for evaluating a health reform – answer these questions

- *What is the reform intervention?* Define the change which is to be evaluated: specifically, what was changed and how it was changed? Is there a detailed implementation plan?
- *What is the immediate target?* Who or what should be different as a direct and immediate result of this intervention?
- *What is the intended immediate effect on this target?* How exactly is the immediate target supposed to be different as a result of the intervention? (What would people do differently or how should the procedure or organisation be different from before the intervention?)
- *What is the ultimate target?* Which group of people should ultimately benefit from the change (e.g. which patients or population)?
- *What is the intended impact on the ultimate target?* What difference is the intervention intended to make for patients or populations?
- *What 'side effects' are to be avoided?* What do we not want to happen as a result of the intervention?

Step 2: define the evaluation perspective

An evaluation cannot discover everything about the reform process and its effects. An evaluation is always partial and limited. The 'evaluation perspective' determines which features of the reform and its effects are examined and the scope of the evaluation. Three things decide the perspective of the evaluation:

Primary evaluation users

Who is the evaluation for and what are they interested in? The more users you try to serve, the less well you will serve any.

Evaluator's perspective

Decide if you will evaluate the change only from the perspectives and interests of the users or include other stakeholders' perspectives (e.g. a public health perspective or the perspective of economically disadvantaged people). The evaluator's perspective also refers to the disciplinary evaluation perspective – to view the reform from an economic, political or other social science perspective with its models and methods.

Criteria for valuing the change

Decide which criteria to use to judge the value of the change. Examples of value criteria are the effect of the intervention on patients and the resources used to introduce the changes. This often involves working with the users to define what is important to them, what they want to know and how they would judge the success or failure of the change. Other examples of criteria by which reforms may be judged are equity in access to services, equity of utilisation of services, quality, total costs, allocative efficiency (are resources allocated according to need?) and technical efficiency (outputs for inputs).

Step 3: define the design

Choice of design

Step 3 involves choosing the design which is most likely to answer the user's questions, given the resources and other constraints on the evaluation. There are four designs which have been used to evaluate health reforms, changes and policies. The most common is a before–after single case design (design 3).

Reform evaluation design 1: describing implementation process and evaluating the process

This design does not look at the effects of the policy, change or reform but describes what was done in implementing it. The evaluator decides which aspects of the implementation to examine and uses interviews and documentation to follow or reconstruct the process. They report on strengths and weaknesses of the process and make explicit the criteria used to assess the process; for example, one criterion might be whether all stakeholder groups were involved. The evaluator may use descriptive case study methods (Yin, 1989) and also draw on an ideal and an actual model of the implementation process to help construct their description.

Reform evaluation design 2: comparing achievements with reform objectives

This design compares the intended goals of the policy, change or reform with the extent to which these are achieved. Using this design to evaluate a decentralised mental health reform would mean finding out the intended goals from documents, deciding which data would allow judgement of the extent to which these goals were met and then collecting and presenting these data. In effect, it means thinking of the goals as the only criterion for valuation of the reform. This may or may not include looking at the ultimate effects of the reform on people with mental health problems or those who are at risk: it would depend on whether this was a stated goal.

Some reforms' intentions do not mention improving health as a goal. If so, this design would not be suitable for some users who had this as a value criterion. The evaluator may also feel that there were missing goals and value criteria which should be used in evaluating the reform, for example the effect on equity. One of the challenges of using this type of design is that goals are often general principles or aspirations and it is not clear which data would give evidence of the extent to which the goals were met. Evaluators usually have to translate goals into what can be measured. Users or other stakeholders may not accept that the measures are valid indicators of goal achievement, so it is wise to discuss these with evaluation users at the planning stage. Note that doing this may help users more clearly to define the objectives, which itself changes the reform.

Reform evaluation design 3: comparing 'before' with 'after'

This design describes the change, reform or policy process but also gathers data before and then after the reform has been proceeding for long enough to have an effect. Which data to collect before and after and the length of time would depend on the value criteria against which the reform is to be assessed: common criteria are costs, efficiency, access, equity, quality and service comprehensiveness.

The data to collect would also depend on the evaluation timescale. If the evaluation results are required soon after the start of the reform (e.g. one or two years), then only some effects might be expected; for example, effects on health providers and organisation.

This design can be used when there are no 'before' data available, because the evaluator could interview different stakeholders and collect their judgements about any before–after differences. The aim is to reach plausible explanations or conclusions rather than statistical probabilistic proof of causality.

Reform evaluation design 4: comparing one site with one or more others implementing the reform

This comparative design gathers data about different sites or areas implementing the same policy, change or reform. It can be used cross-nationally to compare similar types of reform, for example purchaser–provider reforms or market reforms, or within one country to compare different areas. What is compared depends on the evaluation users' interests and value criteria. It usually involves comparing the implementation process at different places and using the comparison to try to discover factors which helped or hindered the speed and depth of the implementation. It may also involve comparing the effects of the reform in different places.

In deciding on a design, consider whether there is the possibility of piloting the policy or reform changes in one area or organisation. This may allow a comparative study. Another possibility is that there may be areas or organisations which have not implemented the reform or where penetration of change has been low or slow and which could serve as a comparison site or a control site or which could allow a 'natural experiment'.

After deciding the design, the evaluator can then plan the timetable for the evaluation and make preparations. This will involve looking ahead to the next step of data gathering and planning how to gather the data needed.

Step 4: gather data

In the following we will assume the design is a single or comparative before-and-after design (type 3 or 4), as these are the most common designs for healthcare reforms. In these designs the following data are required, gathered using the methods described in Chapter 11.

Data about the reform intervention process

The evaluator needs to decide how to gather data about how the policy or reform was implemented in practice (the plans and actual actions). In addition, they need to gather data about which changes were intended and proposed in the reform proposal or instrument.

Data about the environment 'surrounding' the reform

More difficult is to decide which data to collect about the environment or the context of the policy or reform over time. These data are needed to assess whether other factors apart from the intentional change caused any before–after differences discovered.

Data about the effect of the reform on the immediate target

The evaluator needs to decide which before–after data to gather to find out how the target has changed. This depends on what the evaluation user thinks is important in judging the value of the reform (the user's value criteria). How many of these outcomes can be studied depends on the time and resources available and whether data are already collected which the evaluator can use.

Data about the effect of the reform on the ultimate target

Similarly, the evaluator has to decide which before–after data to gather to find out how the ultimate target has changed. The change may take some time to happen, for example effects on population health. It may be necessary to collect data which suggest how the ultimate target might change in the future; for example, data which are a 'proxy' for effects on health such as data about people's access to services which are known to impact health.

Data about other possible effects

All reforms, like treatments, have 'side effects' for the targets and for others. Some are beneficial, some are not. The evaluator needs to decide which data to gather to assess any other possible intended and unintended outcomes of the intervention, bearing in mind the time and resource constraints. One simple method is to ask those deeply involved for their views and if they know of any evidence for these effects.

Note that data can be in two forms: indicators or statistics held in databases, which are reliable over time, or people's subjective perception of events or their subjective assessment of any before–after differences. The 'golden data rule' applies as always: never collect data without checking if there are already data which you can use – check if databases or records or documents have the data you need and are accessible.

Box 3.5: Model of a healthcare reform for identifying the data required for an evaluation

The intervention			Outcomes (intended and unintended)		
Environment of reform and pressures	*Reform aims, instrument and content*	≫ *Reform implementation process* ≫	*Target* of reform instrument	*Effect* on target (short-term outcome)	*Impact* on patients and populations (long-term outcome)

Questions for deciding which design and data-gathering methods to use

- Who is the evaluation for?
- Which decisions or actions could the evaluation inform or make a difference to?
- Which data are readily available and reliable?

Step 5: consider explanations

Having decided the design and collected the data, the fifth step in evaluating a policy or healthcare reform is to consider explanations for the findings. This is the theory-building stage. The main explanations required are about:

- how the intervention was implemented: what helped and hindered the implementation?
- any before–after (or before–later) changes to the immediate targets: apart from the intervention, what other factors might have had an effect on the target and might explain any changes which were

documented (e.g. which features of the target and environment could also explain the outcomes)?
- any before–after (or before–later) changes to the ultimate targets: apart from the intervention, what other factors might explain any changes which were documented to the ultimate target, such as patients?

You cannot assume that the reform caused any outcomes which you have documented. You have to list all the other possible explanations and consider the plausibility of each.

Although this step is towards the end of the six steps, the evaluator needs to be thinking right from the start about how they will make these explanations. You should plan which data to collect to find out how much these factors might explain or cause any before–after differences. It may be possible to compare areas or organisations which have been subjected to the policy or reform with those which have not, or with those where the reform has been slow to penetrate or only partially introduced (e.g. a design type 4 comparison). It is unlikely you will be able to control for these factors, but comparison sites not exposed to the change may allow a limited control.

Step 6: write and communicate evaluation conclusions

The following outlines one way of structuring the evaluation report. Different reports are needed for different audiences, but a full 'master report' should describe the evaluation brief, the methods and the full findings and cover the following points.

1 *The intervention evaluated*: summarise the description of the intended reform or policy. Boxes 3.2 and 3.5 give a quick way to summarise a health reform to explain it to others. Part 4 of the report below is the description of the actual reform process.
2 *Evaluation criteria*: list the criteria used to judge the value of the reform and explain why these criteria were chosen (see Step 2 above).
3 *Type of data gathered*: give a summary list of the type of data gathered, which related to each criterion of valuation.
4 *Describe the process of implementation*: who did what and when?

5 *Summarise any before–after changes* to the targets, ideally in graphs or a visual presentation.
6 *Explain changes*: list factors other than the intervention which might explain the changes documented and present the evidence for and against each factor.
7 *Conclude* with (a) the most significant changes documented, (b) what is the most likely explanation for these changes, (c) how the reform or policy appeared to perform in relation to each criterion for valuation, and the evidence which supports this, (d) the limitations of the evaluation in not gathering data about X, and the limitations of the data and of the design.

Box 3.6: Practical advice for evaluating a healthcare reform

- Focus on specific aspects of the reform or policy and map the causal change chain (Boxes 3.3 and 3.5).
- For a complex multiple-component reform, make separate evaluations of each component and later assess whether there is a mutual reinforcing effect between the components.
- Use the stated aims of the reform and your ideas about likely effects to generate hypotheses to test: this helps to focus on which data/indicators to gather.
- The ideal is the enemy of the good and feasible: realistically assess in relation to the time and personnel you have which data you must collect and which are easily available.
- Ask experts to produce or advise about where the data are and their validity and reliability.
- List which interviewees are accessible (allowing for appointment cancellations and the need to follow new trails as you go).
- Use formal channels to introduce the evaluation and yourself and to get interviewee and expert co-operation (the time saving outweighs the danger of bias and concealment, especially if you 'triangulate' (*see* Chapter 11 on data gathering)).
- List factors other than the reform which are affecting the target, patients and populations and think about how to judge the different effects of the reform (plan the design).

Summary

- Healthcare changes, policies and reforms are more difficult to evaluate than health programmes because the change or reform process is unclear and may itself change over time. 'Environmental' factors such as finance and politicians also change.
- The six steps in evaluating a health policy or reform are:
  1 define the change
  2 define the evaluation perspective
  3 define the design
  4 collect the data
  5 consider explanations
  6 write and communicate the evaluation conclusions.
- How can you evaluate a health policy or reform quickly and objectively? By answering the two questions: what was done and what were the results? (Or if you are planning a prospective evaluation ask what is proposed, what are the likely results and what are the alternatives, including doing nothing?)
- To answer these questions you need to decide which data to collect and how you can find out if the policy or reform or something else caused any results (proving attribution).
- To decide which data to collect, you need to define which criteria are used to judge the value of the policy or reform and which data to collect to inform this judgement.
- To prove the policy or reform caused the results, you need to consider alternative explanations and design the evaluation to exclude these or gather data about them.

Table 3.1: How to assess an evaluation of a health reform or intentional change

	Data (score 0–5)	*Design* (score 0–5)	*Relevance* (score 0–5)
Description of the reform	How good was the description of the actual implementation of the change? (The criterion for a 'good' description is that someone else could repeat it and that the sources are accurate (position and time documented)) How good is the description of the intended changes? (e.g. from official documents) How good is the description of the context to the change? (to enable someone to (a) judge if similar context is present for them, (b) judge whether factors other than the change might have caused any before–after differences which were reported)	How good are the methods used to gather data and to describe the intervention? What is the likelihood of an average professional using these methods being able to create a 'good' description of the implementation process?	How similar is the intervention to one which you are implementing or could implement? How similar is the context to your context?
Effects	Are there before–after data which are valid and reliable? Are other data about possible effects reliable and valid?	Was data gathered about all important and possible effects?	Are these the effects which are of interest in your situation?
Explanation	How probable is it that the before–after differences are due to the intervention?	*Internal validity* Are all other explanations for the before–after differences considered (other than the intervention)? Are these explanations excluded satisfactorily? (e.g. by planning controls before, or by retrospective assessment of their possible influence)	*External validity* How likely are similar effects in your situation if you applied this intervention in your context? (Is it valid to generalise these findings to your situation? What is different and are these differences significant?)

Chapter 4

How to plan an evaluation

If you fail to plan, then you plan to fail.

You plan, and then life happens.

Introduction

Chapters 2 and 3 gave practical steps for evaluating a health service, a programme, a reform or a change. This chapter gives general guidance for planning any type of evaluation. The next chapter considers the practical issues to consider when carrying out an evaluation.

You cannot plan everything, even for a small evaluation. But without a plan which shows the design, data-gathering methods and timetable, the evaluation will surely fail. If you require external finance for the evaluation, then sponsors will require you to propose a plan which shows what you will do, that you have considered other designs and that there are not more cost-effective ways of getting the data. Planning is simply thinking ahead about what you want to achieve and how you will do it. Planning helps you see the different ways of doing things, to decide which approach is possible and the tasks which need to be done. It makes it possible for you to keep track of your progress and to share your thinking with others or for a team to discuss and agree what to do and who will do it.

Evaluation is expensive and time consuming but some evaluations are started without considering what is required for the evaluation to be successful. After reading this chapter you will know how to assess whether a successful evaluation can be made. We give a simple checklist of five questions which you can use when making or managing an evaluation to keep it on track. You will also be able to plan an evaluation using a nine-question guidance tool. If you are financing or managing an evaluation, these tools will help you to assess whether the evaluators have thought through what they will do and whether they are likely to carry out a good evaluation.

Evaluation feasibility assessment (EFA)

Evaluation is worse than useless if it does not make a difference to decisions or make a significant contribution to scientific knowledge. This is because evaluation is expensive and takes time and money away from other activities which could be doing more good. Because of the cost and high failure rate of evaluations, financial sponsors and others are increasingly asking for an evaluation feasibility assessment report before considering a proposal for an evaluation or as part of a proposal for one. Evaluation feasibility assessment (EFA) is made before starting an evaluation in order to decide whether to go ahead or to help plan changes to increase the chances of a successful evaluation.

In one of my first evaluations I looked for the effects of a mental health promotion programme on people in one area. One method I used was to interview a sample of people and it was only then that I realised that the programme had not been reaching most of the people it was intended for. It was too late to redesign the evaluation to look at who the programme had reached or who it had been provided to. The moral of the story: there is no point looking for the effects of an intervention that has not been implemented or has not reached the people it is intended for. An EFA would have revealed the problem and allowed a redesign of the evaluation before it was too late.

The purpose of evaluation feasibility assessment is to decide whether the following conditions for a successful evaluation are present.

- There is a user for the evaluation, who wants information in order to make decisions.
- An 'intervention' such as a service, programme or change does exist and it can be described and separated from its environment.
- Objectives are already defined for the intervention, or objectives could be specified, against which the intervention can be evaluated.
- Relevant data are accessible or can be collected which will help the evaluation user to make decisions.
- The time and resources are available to the evaluators to collect and report the necessary data and to carry out the evaluation.

To some extent an EFA is itself a mini-evaluation. You need to collect data about the intervention so as to be able to describe it, as well as identify the objectives and the types of data about outcomes which can be collected. The EFA report is not just to decide whether to go ahead but provides a valuable basis for planning an evaluation. One way of making an EFA report is to assess whether the five key conditions above are present. A more structured approach is to gather data to calculate a Risk of Evaluation Failure Index (REFI) as shown in Box 4.1.

Box 4.1: The Risk of Evaluation Failure Index (REFI)

This index is a way to check if the preconditions for a successful evaluation are present and helps to give a structure for writing an EFA. The final risk of failure score = (100 − the sum of the scores for each question below).

The intervention

1 Can the intervention be described and distinguished from other activities?
Score 0–5 for how easy it is to draw a boundary around and describe the components of the intervention. 5 is easy, 0 is impossible.

2 Has the intervention been implemented (if the evaluation is not a prospective one)?
Score 5 if the intervention has not been started and the users want to know about the outcomes, 0 if it has been fully implemented.

3 Are there objectives against which the intervention can be assessed or could valid objectives be constructed?
Score 0 for no objectives, 5 for well-specified, easily measurable objectives.

4 Is it possible to gather data to describe how it operates and/or the process of implementation?
Score 0 if not possible or if there are very different and conflicting views, 5 if it is very easy to find out how it operates.

The user's needs, questions and criteria

5 Is it clear which user group the evaluation is for and which of their decisions are to be informed by the evaluation?
Score 0 if it is not clear who the evaluation is for or the decisions they need to make which the evaluation is to inform, score 5 if there is one clear user group and set of decisions.

6 Are the targets of the intervention clear?
Score 0 if there are many different targets and it is not clear which are immediate and which are ultimate targets, 5 if it is clear exactly which people or organisational processes are the target.

---

7 If outcomes are to be assessed, is it clear which outcomes are of interest to the users and what their value criteria are?
Score 0 if it is not clear which outcomes are important to the users, 5 if the users are very clear what they want to know about outcomes to help make their decisions.

The resources

8 Is it clear by when the report is required and which information needs to be in it?
Score 0 if you do not know the timescale or the types of information required. Score 5 if both are specified in writing.

9 Is it clear who will be working on the evaluation, for how much time and their skills?
Score 0 if personnel and the amount of time are not known, 5 if these are known.

The 'quick' guide

Before describing the more detailed guide for planning an evaluation, the following gives a more simple tool. It is five questions which keep an evaluator focused on the information which they need to collect in most types of evaluations. I have found it invaluable, at the start of planning, to use this tool to help think about which data are needed and about the concerns of the evaluation users. To keep me focused I always carry these five questions on a small card when in the field – it is useful when doing an interview and you have lost your questions! A longer list of questions for the field is given in Appendix 3.

Ask these questions when planning and doing an evaluation.

1 What *difference* did it make (outcome)?
Compared to nothing, what would have happened to the target people and to others?

2 Can you *prove* it?
Which data can you gather which show that the difference is real and more than a personal subjective impression?

3 How to make it *better*?
What would make the intervention more efficient and effective and raise its quality? Efficiency is the cost of each item of service and effectiveness is how well the intervention meets people's needs or achieves objectives.

4 Opportunity *costs*?
Could the resources have been better used elsewhere, for other people's needs in other programmes?

5 *Numbers*?
How many, how long, how often, how much?

The discussion below of the more detailed guidance tool explains why these questions need to be answered in most types of evaluations.

The 'nine questions' guide

This planning tool gives a nine question checklist to guide your planning of an evaluation, finishing off with a timetable plan of who will do what and when. The nine questions are listed in summary in Box 4.2. Note that the actual writing of the plan and timetable for the evaluation is the last thing to do – there are a series of questions to answer before one can start planning these practical details. Also planning data gathering comes relatively late after you have clarified which data the users need, your time and resources and the design.

Box 4.2: Nine questions for planning an evaluation – overview

1 *What?*
What are you evaluating (describe the intervention)? Who are the targets? What are the target outcomes (these are the real objectives of the intervention)?

2 *How much?*
Time (by when is the report needed to influence the decisions?). Resources – money and people?

3 *Who?*
Are you doing the evaluation for (your evaluation users/customers)?

4 *Why?*
Which decisions do they need to make which can be better informed (what is the added value of your evaluation)?

5 *Value?*
What is important to them and what do they need to know to help their decisions?

These first five questions give the basis for deciding design, the data needed and the collection methods, timetable and plan, which are covered in the last four 'detail' questions.

6 *Design?*

7 *Data?*

8 *Plan?*
What is our plan – actions and timetable and responsibilities?

9 *Problems?*
What might stop us carrying out our plan? Which changes or possibilities should we explore to improve the evaluation?

The nine question guide is illustrated here with an example of how to plan an evaluation of a quality programme. A quality programme is a set of activities which an organisation carries out to improve quality and includes such things as defining responsibilities, training, project teams and reporting systems.

1   What?

This first question refers to the need to define clearly the intervention to be evaluated, as well as the people or organisation targeted by the intervention, the outcomes expected and the objectives. For evaluations of new programmes or reforms it is often not possible to answer this question precisely; some of the data gathered during the evaluation will be to describe exactly what the intervention is or how it has changed over time.

Define the intervention
- What is the intervention, action, change or 'thing' which you are evaluating?
- What are the component parts?

- Could the intervention change?
- Where will you draw the boundary which separates the intervention from other things surrounding it?

In the example the quality programme is the intervention. The component parts are typically a training programme, a structure of meetings and committees, a process for managing projects and for reporting progress and a quality measurement system. We may define these components by looking at what previous research has found as the key components or by using a model of a quality programme which shows these parts (e.g. Øvretveit, 1999). We can use this to decide which data we need to describe the specific quality programme which we are evaluating and how it changes over time. The most difficult question is the boundary question: what is and what is not the intervention? This is especially difficult to answer for a quality programme because, after the initial stages, the programme should merge into everyday operations.

It is important to remember that this first question directs the evaluator to writing a rough definition; it highlights some of the things which need to be clarified or investigated later in the evaluation.

Define the targets and the outcomes for these targets

- Which people is the intervention for and which needs is it intended to meet?
- In which way will these people be different or behave differently if the intervention is successful?

This second part of the 'what' question refers to who or what are the targets of the intervention. In the example, the immediate targets of the quality programme are health personnel and the final targets are patients.

Define the objectives

- Are there objectives to the intervention? Are objectives written down or in people's heads?
- Decide which objectives you will use for the evaluation.

These questions direct the evaluator's attention to whether the programme has defined objectives and whether these can be evaluated; are they specific enough to allow data to be gathered to decide if the objectives have been met? Often objectives are not well defined and knowing this early in the planning stages helps the evaluator to think about which type of evaluation design to use and whether to spend time working with others trying to define and agree objectives that can be evaluated. Note that the outcomes for the targets are one of the objectives, and may be the only objective.

2 How much?

This question directs the evaluator to thinking about the time and resources for the evaluation. By clarifying this early in the planning stage, the evaluator is able to avoid planning designs and data collection which are not feasible. The five key questions to answer are:

- by when is the evaluation report required?
- how long have you got to complete the evaluation?
- how many people are available, part or full time, and how many person-hours does this add up to?
- budget? How many financial resources for travel and other items will be needed/are there available?
- available data? Which data sources are likely to be easily accessible?

In the example, it may be possible to get help from personnel in the organisation to gather data or help with the evaluation of the quality programme. Clarifying how much time they can give is important for deciding which data can be collected in the time available, as well as clarifying which data are already available.

3 Who?

4 Why?

After clarifying what is to be evaluated and the resources available, the next questions are about who the evaluation is for (the primary user) and how they will use the evaluation. Evaluation is a service for a user and it is important early in the planning to be clear who the user will be and which of their decisions need to be informed by the evaluation.

In the example hospital management personnel are the primary users of the evaluation and their decisions are about how to make the quality programme more cost-effective. Discussion with these users may reveal that they have specific concerns, such as why some quality projects are more successful than others and how to involve physicians in the programme. These discussions can then lead into clarifying the criteria by which the user judges the value of the programme – the fifth planning question.

Common questions which users have are as follows.

- Does it work? (Which criteria do they use to judge this?)
- For whom does it work? (Which perspectives to take when assessing the intervention?)
- Why does it work? (Explain how it works – the causal mechanisms.)
- Does it work in all environments and circumstances? (What environmental factors help and hinder the intervention and which are essential?)

5 Value?

This question directs the evaluator to consider how the evaluation users judge the value of the intervention. Understanding this avoids wasting time collecting data which the users are not interested in. For example, managers judged the value of the quality programme in terms of its immediate effects on personnel morale and the time and money it consumes, as well as in terms of cost savings and solving quality problems. The evaluator will also consider the criteria which others have used in previous evaluations of similar interventions, for example the six criteria described in Chapter 2. Three pertinent questions are as follows.

- What is important to the users about the intervention or its effects?
- By which criteria do *they* judge the value of the intervention?
- Are there other things which you as an evaluator want them to consider?

In the example, the evaluator of a quality programme may decide that they do not know enough about what is important to the users. At an early planning stage they may discuss this subject with managers and agree with them the criteria to use to shape which data will be gathered. In a quality programme which I evaluated, I found that managers wanted to know how much the programme was costing, which projects had been 'successful' and why, and what personnel thought about the programme. No one mentioned specifically whether patient satisfaction or clinical outcomes had been improved, but these were included after I raised the question. The managers were perhaps wiser than I was in understanding how difficult it would be to gather data about these two value criteria.

How certain and detailed do the answers to these first five questions of the 'nine questions' guide need to be? For many evaluations only a rough answer is needed as a basis for planning the evaluation. The questions help to focus on what is important and to highlight areas of uncertainty. They should raise many more questions. The skill is to decide which questions can be answered when the evaluation has started and which need to be answered at this planning stage before the evaluation can start.

6 Design?

This question and the following three help to plan the details of the evaluation. After answering the questions above, the evaluator has enough information to list the evaluation designs which could be suitable and then to choose the design to use. The two main choices about design are about time perspective (retrospective, prospective or concurrent) and about design types 1–6 (discussed in Chapters 8 and 9).

As regards the time perspective, evaluators are often asked to evaluate a health programme or reform after it has started or even finished. It is preferable to plan a prospective evaluation before the intervention starts, but often the best that can be done is a concurrent evaluation.

All the six designs described in Chapters 8 and 9 can be carried out retrospectively, prospectively or concurrently. It helps when planning an evaluation to consider each design as a possible choice and to highlight the advantages and disadvantages of each for answering the user's questions with the resources available. The 'cost of certainty' is a concept which considers how certain the data need to be, for example about outcomes. If the user needs a high degree of certainty then a more expensive comparative control design will be needed (e.g. type 4 or 5 in Chapter 9). Box 4.3 gives a checklist to work through which helps to decide which type of design is best.

Box 4.3: Checklist for deciding design

1 Assess the *stability* and *controllability* of:

	Intervention	Target	Context
Controllable/stable			
Semi-controllable			
Uncontrollable			

In the example, a quality programme changes over time and is not controllable; the same applies to the target personnel and to the environment. This limits the choice of design because it rules out a controlled experiment but a comparison can be used.

---

2 Consider the *user's needs*. By when do they want the results of the evaluation, what are their value criteria and which information do they need? Answers to these questions further limit the choice of design and help to focus on which data are required.

3 *Constraints?* These are the time, resource, skill and data availability constraints which apply to the evaluation. In the example, there were no baseline data about quality so a before–after design could not be used. We had to ask informants to look back and make judgements about the results of the quality programme.

4 *Opportunities?* This question encourages the evaluator to use their creativity and resourcefulness. Are there comparison groups or organisations which could be used as 'controls', for example organisations without a quality programme? Are there data already available which could provide information about the intervention targets or outcomes? Are there personnel in the service who could help gather data or organise access to data or informants?

7   Data?

A common mistake is to collect too much data because you are not sure which you will need. This usually shows that planning was not done properly. Late delivery of evaluation reports is often caused by underestimating the time needed to analyse all the data collected. Data collection takes twice as long as you expect and you should double this time for the time it takes to analyse the data. Remembering this helps you to be realistic and to prioritise exactly which data you must collect.

Working through the questions above helps you to be clear which data are needed to plan data collection. The plan needs to show which data to collect, which data sources could provide these data, how to collect the data and how to analyse and present them. Appendix 4 shows a data-gathering plan which lists the data needed and responsibilities.

The main question is, which data are needed to help the users make their decisions and judge the value of the intervention? Data are usually required:

- for description of the *intervention*
- for description of the *targets*
- about *outcomes* (which type of outcomes? Intended target and unintended? Other outcomes? Before-and-after difference or just people's retrospective judgements?)
- about *alternative or comparable* interventions

- for description of the *environment*
- about *other factors* which could cause the outcomes (other explanations/confounders).

Having listed data sources and collection methods, it is necessary to look again at the time and resources and be realistic about what you can collect and analyse and also ask if you can use data which other people have collected. Chapter 11 discusses different data-gathering methods.

Box 4.4: Guide for deciding which data you need

	Environment	
Intervention	*Target*	*Outcome*
		Short term and long term
Data about the boundary, components and changes	Data about characteristics which might affect outcome	Scope of outcome data to be collected For target, for others

---

8 Plan?

9 Problems?

It is only after answering all the above questions that the evaluator is in a position to draw up a plan. The plan should list the tasks to be done and map out a timetable showing which tasks are to be carried out, over which timescales and who is to be responsible for collecting which data. The plan should also list predictable problems which might affect the plan and the actions necessary to minimise or prevent these; these are discussed in the next chapter.

Box 4.5: Time plan and responsibilities for the eight phases of an evaluation

	June	July	Aug	Sept	Oct	Nov
Phase 1: Initiation	—					
Phase 2: Reviewing knowledge		—				
Phase 3: Preparation	—					
Phase 4: Design planning and choice		—				
Phase 5: Data planning			—			
Phase 6: Data collection and analysis				—		
Phase 7: Reporting					—	
Phase 8: Judging value and deciding action						—

Summary

- Completing an evaluation feasibility assessment report avoids wasting time later, gives a good basis for planning and show sponsors you have thought things through.
- Many evaluations are started without a plan and waste money and time as a result. Two guidance tools for helping to plan an evaluation are the 'quick guide' and the 'nine questions' guide.
- The 'quick guide' asks five questions to help focus on which information is required.
  1 What difference did the intervention make (outcome)?
  2 Can you prove it?
  3 How to make it better?
  4 What are the opportunity costs?
  5 Can you collect numbers about different aspects of the intervention, targets and outcomes?
- The 'nine questions' guide is a more detailed planning method for clarifying the issues before mapping out a plan with a timescale of tasks and responsibilities.
- The first five questions cover what is to be evaluated and for whom.
  1 What is to be evaluated and what are the targets and intended outcomes?
  2 How much time, resources and skills are available?
  3 Who is the evaluation for?
  4 Why? Which decisions do they need to make which can be better informed?
  5 What is important to them (the value criteria they use to judge the value of the programme)?
- The last four 'detail' questions are about:
  6 the design
  7 the data required and how it is to be collected
  8 the timetable plan
  9 the predictable problems and how to minimise these.

Chapter 5

Practical issues and planning

Both the foreseen and the unforeseen will threaten the successful completion of an evaluation. Be open to disasters being a blessing in disguise, and be flexible enough to make the most of opportunities to follow up unexpected discoveries.

Introduction

Ambition is a good thing but evaluators also have to be realistic. The last chapter showed how planning involved recognising what could be done with the time and resources available. Realism also comes from expecting practical problems – the subject of this chapter. Thinking ahead about likely problems does increase the chances of a successful evaluation, but it is not enough. Every evaluation encounters unexpected challenges, such as an evaluation team member becoming pregnant or lost data in a computer crash with no back-up. The many events which throw the study off track call for resourcefulness, creativity, extra time and tolerant family and friends.

Knowing about the likely problems and issues to consider does help, which is the purpose of this chapter: to note common challenges, give practical advice and to look at what needs to be done and by whom during the different phases of an evaluation. 'Forewarned is forearmed' is the theme.

Box 5.1: What I have learned from experience

- The importance of planning, knowing what the evaluation user wants and having clear terms of reference or contract for the study.
- Being flexible and diverting from the plan when necessary. For example, when discovering something unexpected but significant, having the time to follow this up.

- The '*2 *3 law': an evaluation needs twice the money and three times the time that you think it needs, especially if computers are involved.
- The 'p squared law': the more people involved, the more problems, especially in relation to the number of people in the evaluation team and the number of different users of the evaluation whose needs you try to meet (too many cooks and too many diners – cooking for one is easier).
- Generally, the secret of success is to look ahead, get organised and stay flexible.

Practical problems to expect and minimise

The following are common problems which evaluators need to anticipate, try to minimise beforehand and manage when they happen.

'Vague users' unsure of what they want

Often evaluation users or sponsors have not thought about what they want to know from the evaluation or which decisions it should inform. They assume that the evaluator will know which criteria to use to evaluate the intervention. Many evaluators are only too ready to supply their own value criteria, use their favourite methods and assume that they know what is important to the user. The result is that the evaluation findings may not be of interest to the user.

Agreeing with users which information they need is an important early step. The first question to the user is: what is important for the user to know? For example, is it important to know how many of the people who need the service are receiving it? Or how much of the reform has been implemented? The second question is, why? What actions might the user take as a result of the evaluation? The evaluator can propose different criteria for discussion (e.g. the 'six criteria' in Chapter 2) and try to understand exactly which decisions the evaluation should be helping with.

'Gate-crashing users'

When word gets out that an evaluation is being undertaken, many doors close but many also open. Different groups want the evaluation to serve their interests and demand that they are interviewed and that their perspective is represented in the report. Sometimes it is appropriate to represent the full range of views, but limits to the evaluation have to be established if it is to be useful. The evaluation is best designed to meet the informational needs of one or two evaluation user groups. It has to be explained to different interest groups that the evaluation is limited and is only looking at particular aspects. They should either arrange their own evaluation or try to persuade the primary users that their perspective should be included. Sometimes it is politic to give in to requests to be interviewed, but evaluators risk being accused of not representing these views properly in their report.

'After-thought' and 'by tomorrow' evaluation

Many programme, policy and reform evaluations are requested after the intervention has started or as an after-thought or when programme managers remember that an evaluation is a condition for renewed finance. Such last-minute evaluations rule out some designs and data-gathering methods. There are no solutions to this problem apart from decision makers requiring evaluation to be planned in at the proposal stage and before the intervention starts. If the evaluator agrees to a last-minute evaluation, they need to make clear in their negotiations what the limitations will be. They need to report the limitations and the timescale and conditions under which the evaluation was carried out and the other designs and data which were preferable but not possible, because the report may be widely circulated.

No baseline measures, and 'drop-outs'

I was recently asked to evaluate a health programme. One of the criteria was whether more people who needed care were now receiving it. Another was how much the programme had reduced the disease rates in the area. Looking back at the records, I found no data about disease rates before the programme or data which could be used as an indicator of need before the programme. This was a retrospective evaluation and it required me to look for any data about the targets 'before' the intervention started and which could be compared with later data to assess the effect of the intervention. Such 'baseline data' are often not available, which means the evaluator usually has to rely on informants' judgements about the effects. 'Drop-outs' are another common problem, especially for experimental evaluations where some carefully selected target people or organisations are no longer exposed to the intervention or withdraw. This increases the chances of bias because people or organisations who complete the programme may be special in some respect. This can affect the generalisability of the findings. Expect 'drop-outs' and collect data to judge any bias affect they have on the findings.

'Fuzzy' boundaries to the intervention

One of the biggest challenges in our evaluation of the Norwegian total quality management experiment was finding out exactly what was the quality programme which a hospital had implemented (Øvretveit and Aslaksen, 1999). The plans for the quality programmes were not well described and informants gave different descriptions. Our solution was to create from the literature a model of a quality programme and to compare what people had done with this model. This helped us to think of different activities which had not been undertaken before the programme started, such as training or project management, and ask if they were part of the new programme.

A quality programme is a good example of an intervention with boundaries which are 'fuzzy'. The boundary between the intervention and its 'environment' is not clear for most health programmes, and especially so for policies or reforms. Implementation is part of the reform so where do we draw the boundary between the reform and outcomes and other changes? The theory about the actions to implement the reform is different from what you find in practice.

Evaluators should assume that the item which they are asked to evaluate will not have clear boundaries, even if sponsors think that it does. The words used to describe the programme, policy or intervention are only a starting point, which sketches out an area which then needs to be precisely specified for the evaluation to be undertaken. Evaluators should approach all evaluations with a questioning attitude towards where the boundaries of the intervention lie and assume that a key part of the evaluation is to gather data precisely to describe the intervention as it is or was carried out, not as it is intended to be.

'Environmental disorder'

Programmes, policies and reforms are not carried out in the controlled conditions of a laboratory. They exist in the turbulent healthcare environment of elections, changing governments, short-term management contracts, cuts in finance, patient group politics and changing media fashions and obsessions. During a health education programme to reduce heart disease, the government may announce new targets, the media may cover the subject widely when a famous actor has to retire and a new drug may be announced. All this will affect the knowledge, and possibly the behaviour, of the target groups for a local heart disease prevention programme which is being evaluated.

When we are trying to assess the effect of an intervention on a target, we need to assess the extent to which changes in the target were due to these environmental changes or to the intervention. The longer the timescale over which effects are to be assessed, the greater the challenge it is to assess whether the outcomes were due to the intervention. Whilst these changes cannot be controlled, they can be documented by the evaluator and informants can make assessments of the possible impact of these changes on the targets. The evaluator can then describe these confounders and discuss their possible effects.

'Gate-crashing confounders'

The evaluator may be lucky and may know which factors obviously have an effect on the targets, even though these were unexpected. However, during an evaluation new influences which were not expected may begin to have an effect on the outcome variable and make it more difficult to attribute any changes in the outcome to the intervention.

Take the example of a three-year health promotion programme which aims to improve diet and exercise and reduce work stress in a community. One year into the programme the main local employer closes, making 30% of the community redundant, which changes family incomes, gives more 'free time', but increases stress for both unemployed people and those remaining in work. How do the evaluators of the health promotion programme respond to this change? Could or should they have predicted something like this and built such possibilities into the design? Can they use this as an opportunity to do a natural experiment?

'Wobbly' interventions

'Environmental disorder' does not just affect the targets, it changes the intervention. Health programmes, reforms and changes are not like treatments which can be held stable; they are multiple component processes which keep changing whilst the evaluation is being carried out. New personnel may join a programme which is being evaluated and change how the programme is provided. There may be cuts in finance, a sudden crisis which requires a major change or personnel may leave, all of which can significantly change the boundary of the intervention or its component parts.

This is not a problem for action evaluations, which are often undertaken to contribute to the change, but it is a problem for other types of evaluation. Even where experimental evaluations use methods to hold the intervention constant, the chance of unexpected change increases with the length of time of the evaluation. Evaluators should expect the unexpected and consider strategies for detecting changes in the intervention and for deciding how to deal with these changes.

'Ghastly goals' which are unclear or contradictory

One programme which I evaluated had 15 goals on one page. Those which did not contradict each other were general statements of intention about making the world a better place and improving health. The objectives of a programme, policy or reform are usually unclear, conflicting, not measurable without formulating intermediate objectives or there are competing views about objectives. The 'objectives problem' is common and becomes apparent as soon as evaluators give serious thought to how to measure effectiveness or how to judge the 'success' of a service or intervention to an organisation. There are different methods for defining evaluable objectives and for sorting out objectives from unclear statements of goals. One way is to separate higher from lower order objectives by asking 'why?' and 'how?' and to restate objectives in terms of outcomes for the targets, where this is necessary. Appendix 6 gives a model to help structure objectives.

The 'police car' effect

Every child knows that teacher acts differently when the school inspector is there. Who has not driven more carefully when a police car is in sight? Do programme personnel or policy implementers act differently when being evaluated? Do they try to show their work in a favourable light or say what they think the evaluator wants to hear?

I will never forget the two managers of one programme. They openly drew attention to the failures of the programme and wanted me to let them know where improvements needed to be made and to state this clearly in the report. I remember this because it is unusual. These two managers were dedicated to their clients and to improving the programme and sufficiently confident that it would continue to be funded. They were secure in their jobs but were not complacent.

The 'police car' effect is the effect of the evaluation on the personnel and on the intervention being evaluated. People's awareness that something is being evaluated can change their behaviour. They may perform better or worse because they feel that not only are they under scrutiny, but that the evaluation may have good or bad consequences for them. This is not a problem for some action evaluations which aim to create or exploit a 'Hawthorne effect' but for experimental evaluations, it introduces a further variable which is not always possible to control for by 'blinding' targets, providers or researchers.

The 'police car' effect is a different problem from the 'placebo effect', which is the effect on those who are the targets of the intervention of believing that they are receiving an intervention, whether or not they actually receive it.

Missing informants and information

We had travelled for a day over African tracks, which would turn to a mud bath before we left the project. On arrival, we discovered that the project leader whom we needed to interview was absent. All the project documentation was locked safely in her house. Were there any duplicate keys and anyone brave enough to enter?

Yes, we had been expected and yes, there was an explanation. We were suspicious. In fact, we need not have been because this project was the best we saw. By extending our stay we interviewed many more clients, project personnel and community members and later we were able to view copies of key documents held at the central office, including the financial accounts.

There are always missing informants, on leave or not available, and documents and data which have been lost. Anger and suspicion are understandable responses but the African project taught me not to judge too quickly and that there are new insights which can be gained by seeking alternative data sources. It also taught me to write down in the evaluation contract 'requirements about access' to informants and data and about who will be responsible for providing this.

Problems in making valid comparisons

The newspaper picture said it all. A nurse showing a piece of paper to colleagues with exasperation on her face and her hand lifted in an expression of disbelief. The hospital had three times the mortality rates of the other city hospital but was in a deprived area where the emergency room was primary care for many of the homeless and mentally ill living on the local streets. The comparisons had been made without adjusting for the case mix.

Comparison is central to evaluation and all evaluations need to prove that the comparisons made are valid. A problem which sometimes arises is that sponsors want an evaluation of two types of service which appear to be different only in one major respect. I was asked to evaluate whether a new form of teamwork in one primary care centre was better than the traditional one in another centre. However, it was soon clear that the two centres were very different in terms of the number and type of personnel, the physical facilities and the populations served. The services and their environment were in fact very different and con-clusions could not be drawn about differences in costs and outcome being due to the teamwork. Was this why the users were so keen on comparing these centres? Further discussions of problems and solutions in comparative and cross-cultural research can be found in Øvretveit (1998b).

'Distant outcomes' or problems measuring outcome

Many think it is an excuse for lack of results to say that the results of a quality programme or health reform take years to materialise. However, if results do become apparent it is difficult for the evaluator to prove that the results were in fact due to the intervention. Problems often occur in evaluations which consider a multidimensional outcome, such as quality of life, or outcomes some time after the intervention, for example those of a health promotion programme. It may only become clear in retrospect that other variables could have produced the outcome.

One solution is to measure input or process indicators such as whether money was spent or people were recruited and to measure short-term outcomes or outputs such as number of people treated.

'Jar-Jar Binks' team members

Jar-Jar Binks is a character in the film *Star Wars*. He is the extraterrestrial equivalent of an absent-minded hippy, who always gets into trouble. He is loved by children because they can identify with him and because he shows that 'grown-ups' are also capable of making silly mistakes and of being 'organisationally challenged'. Many evaluations are undertaken by teams and often team members are not selected by the team leader or the person responsible for the evaluation. The presence on your team of a 'Jar-Jar Binks' team member will slow down the evaluation, may cause friction and will provide variety and humour, if you have the time and tolerance to enjoy it. Such a member may be able to find out things which other team members could not discover from informants but could damage the team's reputation and will increase the already high number of unexpected problems. Keep them away from computers and sponsors. Do not rely on them to organise transport.

Many of the above problems can be minimised by using the right design, or a flexible one, and by having a detailed practical evaluation plan. Inexperienced evaluators and users need to consider these and other practical problems which are discussed in evaluation texts, but are often better described in the discussion of 'limitations' in different evaluation reports. Checklists for assessing evaluations also alert evaluators and users to possible problems: for example, the 'Economic evaluator's survival guide' (Chapter 8 in Drummond *et al.*, 1987); the 'Review criteria for assessing program evaluations' (Appendix C in DHHSPHS, 1995); the eight methodological criteria given in Daley *et al.* (1992), pp. 138–9; the Standards for Educational Evaluations (JCSEE, 1994); and also HERG (1994) 'Model of research utilisation', pp. 23–7.

Phases in an evaluation: who does what?

Who is responsible for the failure of health personnel to give evaluators the data which they require, or for patients or services 'dropping out' of the evaluation? How can we minimise these problems?

This book emphasises that evaluation is to help people – the users – to decide what to do. For an evaluation to help people to make better informed decisions, there needs to be a link between the users' informational needs, their value criteria and the evaluation design. The users need to be involved in deciding what is to be evaluated and in agreeing value criteria. Later the user draws on findings from the evaluation to decide what action to take.

In the nine phases of an evaluation the user is involved in the earlier and later phases. The evaluation study itself is 'sandwiched' within this larger nine-phase 'evaluation process'. The framework allows the evaluator to prevent the single most common cause of problems: failure to agree the responsibilities of different parties for tasks in each of the phases. The following lists the phases and asks questions which help to define the responsibilities of different parties.

Phase 1: initiation

Who asked for or proposed the evaluation and who is responsible for starting the process: an evaluation user, a sponsor or an evaluator?

Phase 2: reviewing knowledge

The evaluator is usually responsible for this phase of discovering and reviewing what is already known about the intervention or about similar interventions elsewhere. Reviewing involves finding and assessing published research into similar interventions.

Phase 3: preparation

The tasks in this phase are to clarify the time, money and data availability constraints, who the stakeholders are, the users' value criteria and the scope of the evaluation. This is best done by the evaluator in dialogue with the user – a shared responsibility. Preparation involves making an evaluation feasibility assessment, as described in Chapter 4.

Phase 4: design planning and choice

This phase involves answering questions about what exactly is to be evaluated, who are the targets and which outcomes are to be studied (Chapters 2 and 3). These questions are ideally answered through discussion with the users, which then lays the basis for choosing which design is feasible.

Phase 5: data planning

In this phase the tasks are to decide which sources to use, sampling methods and the methods for data collection. In action evaluations the evaluator may involve the users in planning details of which data-gathering methods to use and how to use them.

This phase involves gathering and recording data using qualitative or quantitative methods or both. Everyone needs to be clear beforehand how they will gain access to data and whether health personnel have any responsibilities for collecting or providing data or for giving time to be interviewed.

Phase 6: data-collection and analysis

The tasks are to collect and analyse the data. This phase is usually the sole responsibility of the evaluator, although others may be required to help interpret data.

Phase 7: reporting

The tasks in this phase are to write a report and use different methods to present the findings. Evaluators need to be clear about who will have access to their report and which data they could publish. The users or sponsors may have some responsibilities for publicising results; for example, the report may be only available from sponsors on request.

Phase 8: judging value and deciding action

The users and not the evaluators judge the value of the intervention. They decide what to do by drawing on the evaluation findings as well as other data and by considering the options open to them. Evaluators should clarify at the start whether users expect them to make recommendations and if so, about what. Being clear about this at the outset allows the evaluator to plan how to collect the data they will need to support the recommendations.

Phase 9: evaluator self-review

The last phase is the responsibility of the evaluator, although it may also involve users in giving feedback about how useful they found the evaluation. In this phase the evaluator or evaluation team reviews the lessons for them arising from the evaluation and considers any methodological innovations or improvements which they developed during the evaluation.

Who does what?

Who carries out the tasks and makes the decisions listed for each phase? Is it the evaluator, user, sponsor or health personnel and are some tasks a joint responsibility?

I often find that nurses and doctors do not accept that they should make time to be interviewed and to provide documentation – they are sometimes not told about the evaluation. Evaluators, users, sponsors and others make assumptions about the roles and responsibilities of different parties in an evaluation which may not be justified, especially if they are unfamiliar with the type of evaluation which is being undertaken. If the different parties are not involved in the right way and do not agree their responsibilities, then misunderstandings, problems and conflict are more likely and this can reduce the practical impact of the evaluation.

People who are not evaluators do not know the different tasks. The evaluator is the best person to raise questions about the roles and responsibilities of different parties in the planning phases, to seek agreement before the evaluation gets under way and to continually clarify expectations. The framework of nine phases gives a tool for the parties to agree beforehand who is responsible for what and helps evaluators to clarify their role.

The main parties involved are the:

- sponsor, who may be an external financial sponsor or an internal sponsor who authorises time to be spent on the evaluation
- user, who may also be the sponsor but who is the main person or group who will use the evaluation to decide action
- evaluator(s), who may be one person or a team or more than one team
- health personnel, who may be professionals and managers working in the service being evaluated or who are carrying out a policy or reform which is being implemented and evaluated
- people targeted by an intervention, such as patients or health providers.

Some of the different tasks, responsibilities and roles in most evaluations include the following.

- *The financial sponsor or their agent*: responsible for letting evaluators know when a decision will be made about whether to proceed, for providing finance of agreed amounts at agreed times in agreed ways and for giving agreed amounts of notice for any termination of financing. Sometimes they are responsible for publishing or making the findings available.
- *The steering group overseeing the evaluation*: a group responsible for giving advice and guidance to the evaluator during the evaluation and possibly for receiving and commenting on findings and for helping with reporting. This group may include stakeholders and any rights to direct or over-rule the evaluators on any issues need to be agreed in this group's terms of reference.
- *The evaluators (project leader and staff)*: the limits to their responsibilities need to be defined, together with a timetable for the evaluation and dates for reports and milestones, as well as budgetary and financial responsibilities.

- *Associated helpers (often health personnel)*: in some evaluations there is an agreement that health personnel or others will either co-operate or take an active role, possibly as full members of the evaluation team. The expectations of them and the time for which they are assigned need to be agreed and defined.

Summary

- Planning and technical knowledge are necessary for an evaluation but are not enough to deal with practical problems when they occur. Some problems are common and predictable, but others cannot be foreseen.
- Experienced evaluators try to reduce the chances of the unpredictable damaging the evaluation and have a repertoire of tactics to deal with the more common problems.
- Common problems include: 'vague users' unsure of what they want; 'gate-crashing users' who demand that the evaluation answers their questions after the evaluation has been designed; 'after-thought' and 'by tomorrow' evaluation; no 'baseline' measures and 'drop-outs'; 'fuzzy' boundaries to the intervention; 'wobbly' interventions which keep changing; 'ghastly goals' which are unclear or contradictory; 'environmental disorder' where the context changes; the 'police car' effect; missing informants and information; problems in making valid comparisons; 'distant outcomes' or problems measuring outcome; 'gate-crashing confounders'; and 'Jar-Jar Binks' team members.
- Many practical problems can be prevented by the evaluator clarifying their role and other parties' responsibilities in each of the nine phases of the 'evaluation process'.
- Users have a more active role at the beginning and end of the evaluation process of initiation, reviewing knowledge, preparation, design planning and choice, data planning, data collection and analysis, reporting, judging and deciding action, and evaluator self-review.

Part 2

Evaluation tools

Chapter 6

Concepts for making sense of an evaluation

Introduction

Health professionals, managers and policy makers now need to be 'evaluation literate'. As well as being held accountable for the results of our decisions, we are also being held accountable for knowing about recent evaluation reports. We are expected to understand an evaluation report and to decide the implications for patients, populations, health-care organisations and policies.

It is impossible to keep up with all the evaluation research in one field, but every professional is expected to be aware of the main reports summarised in their professional journals. Some reasons why we do not are because we do not have the tools quickly to understand an evaluation report, assess it and decide what it means for our work and organisation.

This chapter presents conceptual tools and a checklist for making sense of an evaluation report. The nine concepts are listed in Box 6.2 below. Many professionals find that this toolkit saves time and helps them critically to assess a report. It makes the knowledge basis of our profession more accessible and gives a framework for designing our own evaluations.

One tool is a box diagram, which is a way of drawing a picture of the thing which was evaluated and of the evaluation design. It shows the intervention and the targets 'going through' it. This picture is a fast and powerful way to summarise an evaluation. Another even simpler way to draw an evaluation – the EITO model – is also described. The next chapters use these ideas to show the different evaluation designs for evaluating services, policies and changes to health organisation.

After reading this chapter you will be able to:

- quickly understand an evaluation you read and its implications by using the nine concepts to analyse it
- speak the language of evaluation, which is based on these nine concepts, and be able to discuss evaluations with others
- quickly see the strengths and limitations of a particular evaluation
- use evaluation concepts to design your own evaluation.

An example evaluation is used to illustrate the concepts, which is summarised in Box 6.1. This is an evaluation of a work-based active rehabilitation programme for people with shoulder and neck disorders. It compared this service to a traditional primary care service for people with this condition.

Box 6.1: Example evaluation of a rehabilitation programme (from Ekberg *et al.*, 1994)

Is active multidisciplinary rehabilitation more effective than traditional primary care rehabilitation?

An active multidisciplinary rehabilitation programme provided by an occupational health unit was compared to a traditional primary care rehabilitation service in one area of Sweden. The patient groups compared were working people with neck or shoulder disorders who consulted physicians in each service over a three-month period. Patients were selected for both groups if they had not been on continuous sick leave for the disorder for more than four weeks before or did not have other serious health problems.

One group received eight weeks of active multidisciplinary rehabilitation which involved physical training, education, social interaction and workplace visits. The primary care control group were given physiotherapy, medication and rest or sick leave, as thought necessary by the physician.

The outcomes measured in both groups were the average number of days of sick leave for two years after the rehabilitation. Self-reports of symptoms and pain on a questionnaire were gathered before and at 12 months and 24 months. A short version of the Sickness Impact Profile was used before and at 12 months to measure health-related behaviour such as mobility, social behaviour and recreational pastimes. Also at 12 months after the rehabilitation, patients were asked about changes in the workplace.

The findings were that there was no significant difference in outcome between the two groups. However, changes in the workplace such as new tasks or a new workplace were associated with decreased sick leave. This effect was found for both groups and was independent of the type of rehabilitation programme which they received.

Box 6.2: Evaluation concepts – summary

1 *User*: the people for whom the evaluation was designed, to help them make a more informed decision.
2 *Value criteria*: what is important to the user of the evaluation, for their decision or action.
3 *Intervention*: the intervention is the action (e.g. service, project) or change (e.g. a policy, reform) whose value is to be judged.
4 *Target*: the person, population, organisation, process or thing to be changed by the intervention.
5 *Outcome*: any results of the intervention or action – what 'comes out' of the action taken.
6 *Objectives* (of the intervention/change): the difference which the intervention is intended to make to the target. The intended outcomes for the target people.
7 *Confounder*: what confuses or can 'mix with' the intervention or the targets, so that we cannot be certain if it was the intervention or something else which caused the outcomes.
8 *Control*: what is done to hold confounders constant or to exclude them from having an influence.
9 *Data gathering*: the data collected about the outcome and about the intervention and its environment.

Concept 1: the evaluation 'user' or 'customer'

These are the people for whom the evaluation was designed, to help them make a more informed decision. Examples of users of evaluations are health professionals, managers, patients and policy makers such as politicians and their advisors. Who are the primary users of the example evaluation report about an 'active' and a 'traditional' rehabilitation programme above? Is it managers, professionals or others? A clue to deciding who the primary users are is to look at which measures were used and which data were collected. These include data about sick leave, about symptoms and pain and about the impact of the sickness on health and lifestyle. Who is interested in these data and which decisions could these data help to make? We can guess that the main users are professionals and managers.

The key question is, who is the primary user? Many people read and use evaluation reports, but the 'users' are the people for whom the evaluation was designed. Managers and professionals will use an evaluation of a home care service for people returning home from hospital after surgery. But so will patients' organisations who have particular concerns about the patients' experiences and how the service supports the patients' carers. The more users which an evaluation tries to serve, then the less well it serves any. Many evaluations are inconclusive because they try to serve too many different users and different stakeholder perspectives. The design becomes confused and there are not enough resources to collect all the different data which are required for the different interest groups. One reason that many evaluations are not acted upon is that they are not designed for and with specific users, to take account of the information which they need for their decisions. This is why this book proposes a user-focused approach. The primary user can also be other researchers or the 'scientific community'.

The evaluator serves, but is not a servant of the user.

Concept 2: value criteria

The value criteria are what is important to the user of the evaluation. Examples of criteria for judging the value of an intervention are: that it cures symptoms, that a person lives longer, that the experience of undergoing a treatment is not painful, a training programme is not boring, that there are no harmful side effects, the amount of resources used by the intervention, or how easy it is for people to carry out a treatment or reform.

What criteria were used to judge the value of the rehabilitation treatment? Looking at the outcome measures, we would assume that the criteria of valuation were ability to work (as indicated by sick leave claims), reduction of pain and return to previous activities and functions. How did the evaluators decide these value criteria? Probably by thinking about what is important but also about what was measurable in practice and also by looking at what other researchers had measured. We do not know if they consulted users but they may have imagined what would be important to them. Many research evaluations are oriented towards using the measures and value criteria which researchers have used previously. This is because the main users may be other researchers and because contributing to knowledge means relating the research to previously published studies.

Does a user-focused approach to evaluation mean that the evaluator only employs the user's value criteria to judge the value of an intervention? There are three answers, all of which are 'no'. First, the main users may be the scientific community whose main interest is building a disciplinary knowledge base. Depending on who pays for the research and the evaluator's independence, the evaluator may use criteria which have been used in earlier published studies. This does not mean that these criteria are not relevant to other users such as patients, professionals and managers, just that these criteria are not the primary ones and when choices have to be made about the scope of the evaluation, values and measures used in previous research will take priority.

The second answer is that practising users such as managers who sponsor an evaluation often want the evaluator to find out how other people value the intervention and to use these value criteria in assessing it. Managers may want evaluators to find out what patients feel is important about a service to be evaluated. Medical research is increasingly taking into account the patients' perspective when deciding the criteria by which to value a treatment or service. Quality assurance evaluations or audits use value criteria such as patient satisfaction, clinical outcomes and service accessibility.

The third answer is that a user-focused approach does not mean that the evaluator cannot suggest to users criteria by which to value the intervention. They may propose criteria from previous research or their own. For example, managers might not think of equity as a value criterion for evaluating a health reform but the evaluator may propose it and argue for its inclusion.

Value, like beauty, is in the eye of the beholder.

The problems arise when users and sponsors do not accept the evaluator's suggestions and want to limit the scope. The evaluator then has to decide if they are willing to accept this limitation and the criticisms which may be made by others. But limiting the scope is necessary and helpful, which raises another more common problem. This is that the evaluator adopts too many criteria for valuing the intervention – the user's criteria, some from previous research and their own – which makes design and data collection almost impossible. The fewer the users and the value criteria, the easier the evaluation. All evaluations are limited and partial; the question is whether the evaluation describes honestly, and proudly, these limitations and is self-critical.

One approach is to involve all stakeholders in a process for listing and then agreeing a limited set of criteria. This gives the evaluation more credibility with stakeholders, can help to gain access to data and also increases the chances of the findings being implemented. The criteria listing process can form part of a longer process which involves stakeholders later in collectively discussing actions which should follow from the evaluation; it can give a model of an implementation process.

The main point is that being clear about the user's value criteria helps the evaluator to focus on which data to collect so as to provide the user with the information which they need for their decisions. It is also important to limit the number of criteria to be used to make the evaluation manageable. This may require working with users to help them clarify their value criteria, which takes time but will increase the utility of the evaluation.

Box 6.3: A simple EITO diagram of an evaluation

   Environment

Intervention → **Target** ⟶ **Target outcome**

Action   *People or*   *How are they different?*
                  organisations?   *Short term?*   *Long term?*

Concept 3: intervention

The intervention is the action (e.g. service or project) or change (e.g. a policy) whose value is to be judged. In the rehabilitation example the intervention was a 'multiple component' rehabilitation programme of physical training, education, social interaction and workplace visits, which was compared with another intervention – the traditional primary care treatment.

Intervention means 'to come between' what otherwise would have happened (Latin *inter-venere*). In one sense this is an inaccurate word to use for the thing we are evaluating, because the purpose of the evaluation is to see if the thing does make a difference: calling it an intervention assumes that it does. A policy or health reform is an intervention in a sense, but a better term might be a change or an action or a process of change.

In healthcare, we evaluate many different things.

1   Treatment and assessment methods.
    - Single item (e.g. a pharmaceutical, breast cancer screening)
    - Multiple item (e.g. an alternative holistic cancer treatment)
2   Health programmes or services (e.g. a primary healthcare service, a vaccination programme)
    - Serving many people over time (same patient group or many different groups)
    - Giving different types of treatment, education or other interventions
3   Interventions to organisation or reforms, for example a new method of financing (e.g. from payment per diem to by diagnostic-related groups or by capitation), a hospital merger, a training programme for nurses, a quality programme or a healthcare reform (large scope intervention).
4   Health policies or health education/promotion: for example, a policy to increase exercise or 'healthy living' or a 'healthy city' policy.

Some changes or reforms are simple, but some are complex, such as the UK market reforms of the early 1990s (Robinson and Le Grand, 1994). The intervention may be stable or it may change. The variety of interventions and changes which we need to evaluate means that we need to be able to use different methods.

> *To define something is to decide the limits of it. It is not always easy to separate the boundary of an intervention from its environment and from its effects.*

Tools for defining an intervention or change

There are three features of an intervention or change which are significant for the evaluator: the specifiability of the intervention, the stability and the timespan. For example, a drug treatment is easy to describe and to specify the amount and how it is taken. It is stable (does not change) and we can describe the period of time over which it was taken.

Specifiability is how easy it is to describe the intervention. Stability means that the intervention does not change or that we can hold it constant. The timespan of the intervention is whether it started and finished in a short time or a long time, such as many health promotion programmes. Some interventions may be continuous and evolving such as many quality programmes and health reforms. We can describe the rehabilitation example as of average stability and specifiability and of medium-term timespan compared to other health programmes.

Because it is so important clearly to define the intervention, the following gives tools to help readers of an evaluation to understand exactly what was evaluated and to help evaluators to specify the intervention when planning their study.

Components?

These are the different parts or actions of an intervention. Both the active rehabilitation and the primary care rehabilitation in the example had different components. Breaking down an intervention into its component parts helps to describe it.

Change?

This question considers whether the intervention changes during the evaluation. Complex interventions, such as most health reforms, inevitably change over time. Does the report describe the change? How will an evaluator collect data about the change and how will they take this into account when they make their report? In the example, the report did not describe any significant change to the rehabilitation programmes during the period they were given to patients.

Boundary?

The third question covers where the boundary lies between the intervention and its surroundings or 'environment'. The boundary separates the action which is evaluated from other things and has to be clearly defined by saying what is and what is not the intervention. In the example, the rehabilitation programmes were separated from other things like a change to work task or place of work.

Why are these three features – the components, change and boundary – significant? Because these are variables of the intervention which affect which design and methods the evaluator can use, a point to which we return in the next chapter. We will also see how to represent the intervention by drawing a box diagram. This shows the components of the intervention inside the box, and the box boundary separating the intervention from its 'environment'.

The most common shortcoming of evaluation reports is not clearly describing the intervention or change which was evaluated. This makes it difficult for the reader to understand exactly what was evaluated or to repeat the intervention and get the same results. From the example, can we understand exactly what was evaluated? We usually need to look beyond a summary to the full report to find a more detailed description of the intervention.

Concept 4: target

The target of the intervention is the person, population, organisation, process or other thing to be changed. The people who were receiving the rehabilitation services were the targets in the rehabilitation example. But does the report describe characteristics of the targets which may be important? For example, how long they had a neck or shoulder disorder before they received the intervention or their age and sex? These characteristics may affect how the patients respond to the treatment and knowing this helps the reader to judge if they would get similar results with their patients, population or organisation. Other data about the targets are also needed, such as how many of the original group do not complete the treatment ('drop-outs') and why.

The report gives more details about the targets: 53 people received the active rehabilitation and 40 the traditional programme; all were within the 18–59 age group and had been employed in their present occupation for at least two months. The drop-out rate for those who did not complete the treatments was 13% for both groups. We also learn from a table the number in each group who were smokers, their type of employment, how many have children and other details which were not significantly different for both groups.

The targets for most services, health programmes and training programmes are easy to describe and collect information about. But the targets of some health policies and health reforms are more difficult to describe. What is the target of a decentralisation reform? Is it the organisations at different levels of the health system? Targets are always people, but sometimes it helps to think of an organisation or a process as a target, especially when evaluating a change to organisation or a new financing method. The main question is, who or what does the intervention aim to change? For a health reform it may be necessary to separate immediate targets (e.g. health professionals) from ultimate targets (e.g. patients or the population).

An intervention does not just affect the targets. The example evaluation only collected data about the target patients and did not collect data about how carers, employers or health providers were affected by the programme – the difference it made for them. The next section about outcomes distinguishes the outcomes for the targets from the outcomes for other people.

Concept 5: outcome

The outcome of an intervention is what 'comes out' of it or the results. It is the difference which the intervention makes for the targets, but also for other people. The outcomes reported in the rehabilitation example are sick leave, pain symptoms and activities and functions for the patients which are measured in different ways. The example does not report the effects of either programme on family members, health personnel, work colleagues or employers. Neither does it report how many resources are used, which is one outcome described in economic evaluation studies.

Most evaluations concentrate on finding out if the intervention does have the effect which is predicted or expected. But there may also be both unintended and undesirable outcomes to an intervention. All interventions have 'side effects'. Some evaluations gather data to check for possible side effects, but few gather enough data to discover unpredictable or unexpected outcomes, especially those which only appear over a longer term, such as complications 10 years after hip replacements. The 'scope' of the outcome data refers to how broadly the evaluators look for different types of outcomes – not just those which are intended for the targets. 'Scope' refers to how 'wide' the evaluation data-gathering net is cast and the timescale over which the data are collected. A wide scope will be more likely to capture unintended outcomes.

Points to remember

- Only one small part of the outcome can be measured – usually one or two outcomes for the targets.
- The scope of outcome data collection refers to the number of types of outcome data (breadth) and the timescale over which data are collected.

Table 6.1: Outcomes for a drug treatment

	Short term	Long term
Target outcome		
Intended (predicted?)	Symptom relief	Return to work
Unintended – Good	Lower blood pressure	Sustained
– Bad	Nausea	Dependence
Other outcomes (not for the target)		
Intended (predicted?)	Time and money consumed	Money-saved
Unintended – Good	Simpler to administer	More savings
– Bad	Supplier raises prices	Personnel misuse the drug

- The decision about which outcome data to collect is influenced by the evaluation users' values (defined as the evaluation criteria), the intended outcomes and predictions about what effects the intervention might have.
- Outcomes are predicted by a theory about how the intervention might work (the 'mechanism' or 'causal chain').

Concept 6: objectives

One way to evaluate something is to assess to what extent it achieved its objectives. For example, did the rehabilitation programme in the example achieve the objectives set for it? This depends on having a clear statement of the objectives of a service, programme, policy or reform. No objectives were stated for the programme in the evaluation report, but we could imagine that the objectives were related to the criteria of valuation: ability to work, pain relief and return to function.

In my experience it is unusual to have clear and evaluable statements of the objectives of an intervention. For example, one service had as one of its objectives:

> Our objective is to give five sessions of physiotherapy as soon as possible after referral by the physician.

This statement does have a specific and measurable aim, but it is not an objective in the specific sense defined here. It is an action, not an objective, because it does not define the target people or an intended outcome for them – how they should be different. An objective is an intended outcome for the target people. For example, that 'after five sessions of physiotherapy patients should report 50% less back pain and 30% return to function as defined by the function measure.' An objective is the difference the intervention is intended to make to the target.

If not defining the intervention clearly is a common shortcoming of evaluation reports, then not defining clear objectives for actions is the most common shortcoming of health managers and policy makers. People often say what they will do in terms of activities, not what they want to achieve in terms of results. Or they mix actions and outcomes when writing objectives. However, stating activities is a good first step towards defining objectives because we can then think about what difference our activities will make for the targets of the activities. One method of doing this is to ask 'Why?': 'Why do we want to give five sessions of physiotherapy as soon as possible after referral?'

Evaluators often have to take badly defined objectives and redefine them so that they can be evaluated. This may involve working with service providers to construct a definition of the objectives of the intervention. These concepts help to write better objectives.

Intervention → Outcome for the Target → Measure of Target Outcome
(ACTION)   (RESULT)   (INDICATOR)

Evaluators usually have to separate lower and higher objectives, then separate actions from results and then decide which measures/data to collect about results. The step outcomes hierarchy model illustrated in Appendix 6 shows how to do this.

Concept 7: confounder

Confounders are other things which might cause the results. Confounders are what confuses or can 'mix with' the intervention or the targets so that we cannot be certain if it was the intervention or something else which caused the outcomes. In the example, just three confounders which could 'mix with' the rehabilitation programme were the enthusiasm of the personnel to show that the programme was effective, patients feeling that they were getting a special service and patients being treated differently by their employers because they were in the programme.

All evaluations have to wrestle with the problem of 'attribution'. How do we know that the intervention caused the result and not something else? We can never be certain but we have to try to reduce the plausibility of other explanations. When reading an evaluation we should imagine all the other things which could explain the results, apart from the intervention, and then judge whether the evaluators took these into consideration.

One way to exclude confounders is through designing the evaluation to do so. An example is to have two similar groups of people – and one group does not get the intervention but are in all other respects similar to those that do. Another way is to ask informants for their judgements about what came out of an intervention, then to ask them what else could also explain those outcomes and then ask them to assess how much these things could have accounted for the outcomes.

Many evaluations do not just try to find out if the intervention made a difference, but also how it worked. They try to identify the causal mechanisms and the factors which are essential for the intervention to have an effect. For example, how do the different components of the rehabilitation programme work to produce the outcomes? Which factors of the environment are necessary for the programme to operate – the necessary environmental conditions? Knowing this helps evaluation users to decide if they can replicate the intervention and the results.

It may be necessary to exclude confounders to be sure that an intervention does have effects, but we also need to understand the positive and negative effects of confounders. One way to do this is to use a system model to identify which environmental factors are important and the causal mechanisms which operate in and outside the intervention process (Box 3.3). The type of explanation given in many social research and action research evaluations (Chapter 14) is to find the ways in which environmental factors interact with the intervention and target to produce the outcome (the EITO pattern).

Box 6.4: The EITO system model to identify necessary conditions and mechanisms which produce the outcome

Environmental factors
(*These affect the target and intervention*)

Target → Intervention process → Outcome

Environmental factors

The intervention produces the outcome, but only in interaction with its environment, which also interacts with the targets.

Concept 8: control

Control is what evaluators do to hold confounders constant or to prevent them from having a possible influence. In the example the evaluators used an intervention group of patients and a control group. The idea was to try to exclude such things as changes in the local area and other factors which could affect outcome by comparing two groups who were different only in that one received the intervention and one did not. This is a common way to introduce control, as is comparing one area or organisation which was subjected to a change with another similar one which was not.

Is it possible to control all confounders? Practically, no, but also because we often do not know which factors and characteristics could also have an influence. What we can do is to try to increase our certainty that only the intervention causes the outcomes and that the probability of the outcomes is greater than chance. Randomisation of targets goes a long way towards excluding such unknown factors but may not be possible, as we will see in coming chapters.

Often health programme or reform evaluations are not able to control confounders and instead they seek to understand which factors affect the performance of the intervention. They may try to build an EITO model of the intervention and its environment to understand these factors (Box 6.4) or use comparison organisations or areas.

Concept 9: data gathering

In many programme or reform evaluations we do not just need to gather data about outcomes. We need to understand how the outcomes were produced: what was it about the intervention, the environment, the target people or organisations which caused these outcomes? We need to build a picture of the interaction between environment, targets, the intervention and the outcomes and we need data about each of these.

Data gathering refers in part to the tools we use to gather data about outcomes; these are often measurement methods such as questionnaires given to people before and after or some physiological measure. We also need data about the targets' characteristics, such as people's age and sex or an organisation's size in order to assess whether other things apart from the intervention could explain outcomes. Sources such as patient records or other documents are used for this.

To understand how the intervention or change works, we also need data about the process of how the intervention is carried out. We need to study what was done in the health programme or health reform. We also need data about the environment – about what 'surrounds' the targets and the intervention and which may help or hinder the intervention. For example, do the people live in an area of high unemployment or are there financial or other changes happening locally which could affect how the intervention works on the organisation? Chapter 11 describes the main data-gathering methods used in evaluation.

Table 6.2: Data-gathering methods

	Environment	Targets	Intervention process	Outcomes
Patients as targets	e.g. unemployment	e.g. age, sex, income	e.g. what did programme personnel do?	e.g. lower blood pressure, patient health reports
Organisations as targets	e.g. financing, community support for a merger	e.g. size, culture, personnel, morale	e.g. how the merger process was carried out	e.g. whether the organisation's merger was successful

Summary

- Healthcare professionals need to be evaluation literate and to be able to read an evaluation and decide whether they or their organisation should act on the findings. The concepts covered in this chapter enable you quickly to make sense of an evaluation.
- The concepts are: the user (of the evaluation); their value criteria; the intervention; the target (of the intervention); the outcomes; the objectives of the intervention; confounders; control; and data-gathering.
- Evaluations are to help people make better informed decisions. To do this evaluators need to know what is important to users for their decisions – the users' value criteria.
- The more users which an evaluation tries to serve, then the less well it serves any. Many evaluations are inconclusive because they try to serve too many different users.
- A precondition for a good evaluation is to be able to limit it. Evaluators need to limit their evaluation and to explain the limits. They should aim to be certain about a little rather than uncertain about a lot.
- A common mistake made by evaluators is failing clearly to describe the intervention which they evaluated. Managers and policy makers often make the mistake of defining objectives as broad aims or activities, not as outcomes.
- The EITO system model shows how the environment, intervention and targets interact to produce outcomes.

Chapter 7

Evaluation design

Introduction

This and other chapters of Part 2 give tools – concepts, models and methods – for understanding an evaluation. The tools help you to make sense of an evaluation and see its limitations. The tools help to assess which conclusions are justified by the evidence and also help you to design and plan an evaluation.

This chapter introduces evaluation design: the next two chapters describe the six types of design most often used in healthcare. An evaluation design shows the main features of an evaluation study in note form. It is a model including the intervention which is evaluated, the targets of the intervention, the timescale and the data collected. The model does not show the details of data-gathering methods or the timetable and practical plans – these are discussed in Chapters 4, 5 and 11.

Drawing a picture of an evaluation design is the best way to summarise it. I am continually reminded of this in my teaching: I often have groups of 30 students from up to 11 different countries and we are able quickly to communicate reports we have read or plans for evaluation studies – a picture tells a thousand words and speaks across languages. It forces you to pick out the main features from the details of an evaluation report you are reading or one you are planning. Drawing and identifying the type of design also helps you see the most important strengths and limitations of a study. If you can't draw it, you don't understand it.

After reading this chapter you will be able to:

- describe the time perspective of an evaluation: whether the evaluation is made retrospectively, prospectively or concurrently
- use the 'box' model to draw the design
- describe the differences between the six main types of design
- use the 'NIPOO' model to define the intervention, targets and outcomes.

Chapter 10 explains how to choose the best design and how to assess an evaluation study so as to decide whether to act on it.

Design: time perspective

The time perspective of the design is whether the evaluation 'looks backwards' after the intervention has started (retrospective) or 'looks forward' before the intervention (prospective) or is carried out whilst the intervention is happening (concurrent or contemporaneous). Evaluators are often asked to evaluate a health programme or change after it has started and do not have a choice about this aspect of design. Which of the following describes the time perspective of the rehabilitation evaluation example (Box 6.1) shown in the last chapter? This example compared a work-based rehabilitation programme with a traditional primary health-care programme.

Retrospective evaluation

Intervention ←——————— Evaluator looks back at what happened

Starts 2001   Finishes 2002   Start evaluation in 2003

An example is an evaluation of the impact on workers' health of a new form of work organisation, when the evaluation is made two years after the new work organisation was implemented. The evaluation 'looks back' using occupational health records and interviews with workers and managers. Another example is an evaluation of a health reform three years after by using administrative data and questioning different stakeholders about their assessment, in retrospect, of the impact.

When should or could evaluators use a retrospective design? This depends on whether the evaluator can satisfactorily reconstruct what happened. Are there documentation or data collected in the past which are sufficiently valid and reliable to answer the evaluation questions? In social research and action evaluations, it also depends on whether informants are available and on their memory. Triangulation is a useful method for checking data from one source with data from another source. In this way it is possible to build up a more complete picture and to identify conflicting data which needs further investigation. This technique is discussed in Chapter 11.

Prospective evaluation

Plan data gathering and controls *before* ⟶ The intervention

Start planning the evaluation in 2002   Start intervention in 2003

Many medical research evaluations are prospective. Most prospective designs follow the model of a scientific experiment and test predictions. The intervention is viewed as an experiment and the design sets out to test the intervention as if it were a hypothesis: 'We predict that this health programme will have no benefit.' The evaluator is able to think ahead about all the possible confounders and then design the 'experiment' to exclude the most likely and serious events which could later make it difficult to be sure if the intervention caused the outcomes. Prospective designs allow controls to be planned, rather than looking back and trying to assess the effect of different events, such as the effect of key personnel leaving a health programme.

It is common for evaluators to be asked to carry out evaluation retrospectively. The data which are available and people's memories often leave much to be desired and it is difficult to identify, control for and assess the effects of confounders. For these and other reasons a prospectively planned evaluation design is preferable and should be 'built into' any programme or policy before it is implemented. The rehabilitation evaluation described in the last chapter used a prospective design, which allowed the evaluators to select patients and control for patient characteristics before giving the service. It also allowed them to have some control over the stability of the experimental and the traditional rehabilitation programmes and to collect data about whether these changed in any major respect during the evaluation.

Not all prospective evaluations are experimental. A feasibility evaluation or option appraisal 'looks forwards' and is done before an intervention. An example is a feasibility evaluation of a post-surgery recovery hotel (the proposed 'intervention') to help patients' transition to living at home. The evaluation gathers data about possible costs and benefits and patients' views and compares this proposed 'intervention' with the alternatives. If the data gathered suggest that the costs of the 'half-way hotel' outweigh the benefits, then management may decide not to go ahead with it.

Concurrent or contemporaneous evaluation

It is possible to gather data while the intervention is happening and complete the evaluation before the intervention finishes. This design can be used to give feedback to decision makers who are implementing a reform, programme or policy to allow them to make adjustments. An example is the action evaluation of the quality programmes in six Norwegian hospitals, where the evaluators reported data about the progress of the programmes to six-monthly meetings of representatives from each hospital (Øvretveit and Aslaksen, 1999).

Strengths and weaknesses

'We had to do the evaluation with no baseline data' is a common complaint of many evaluators. A prospective design is preferable for all types of evaluations because it makes it possible to decide which data to collect and which controls to design-in. In practice, evaluators often have to use a retrospective design, where the evaluator is dependent on already collected data and people's memories and is less able to control for confounders. A retrospective design could have been used for the evaluation of the rehabilitation programmes if the patient records and documentation for both programmes met research evaluation standards. However, it would not be the optimum design because, if there are enough patients, then patient matching for the two groups is not as good as randomisation, for reasons explained in Chapter 9. Concurrent evaluation design can be useful if decision makers want information quickly. The evaluator is able to build up a picture from different data sources and to follow up conflicting data at the time, rather than retrospectively. But such designs cannot give data about outcomes unless they are carried out for some time.

There are many other ways of describing approaches to evaluation, but these are not designs as such. For example, evaluations can be described in terms of their purpose: a 'formative' evaluation is one carried out to help form the intervention and any of the three designs above could be used for this purpose. A 'summative' evaluation is carried out after the intervention to 'sum up' what happened. 'Process' evaluations are carried out to concentrate on the process of programme or policy implementation, in contrast to 'outcome' evaluations which look at impact. Chapter 14 further discusses different perspectives and philosophies in evaluation.

The 'box' model for drawing an evaluation design

One of the quickest ways to make sense of an evaluation, or to design one, is to draw a diagram of it. The simplest way to do this is to use the 'EITO' model described in the last chapter (Boxes 6.3 and 6.4) and to show on a diagram the intervention, then the target and then the outcome. This is the best method for complex or difficult-to-understand policies and changes.

The box diagram method (Figure 7.1) shows the intervention – for example, a rehabilitation programme – as being inside the 'box' and the people exposed to the intervention as 'passing through' the box. The environment of the intervention 'surrounds' the box. Usually we examine the effect which the intervention has (the difference it makes) and concentrate on looking for the predicted or the intended outcomes.

What is in the box?

This question refers to the box in Figure 7.1 and is the first question to answer in understanding an evaluation report. The box represents the boundary of the intervention and the different components are written in the box. The length of the box is the time over which the targets are 'exposed' to the intervention.

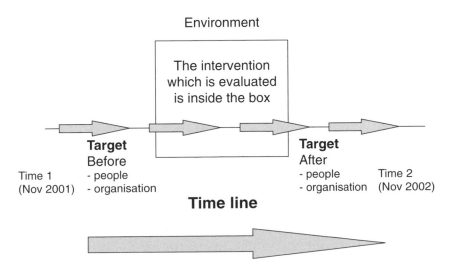

Figure 7.1 Basic 'box' diagram for drawing an evaluation.

The 'box boundary' defines what is and is not evaluated. In the example given in the last chapter, the multidisciplinary occupational health rehabilitation programme is inside the box and we would write inside the box the different components of the programme: physical training, education, social interaction and workplace visits. Other things which happened during the same period are 'environmental factors' which are not evaluated and are outside the box. We could write outside the box changes which could affect the target such as 'change in work task', 'change in workplace'. We could also write outside the box any changes which could have affected the intervention such as a cut in funding for the programme, but no such changes were described in the report.

If you are not clear exactly what was evaluated in a study (the intervention), then you cannot understand the study. This may be because the study was poorly described in the report or it was a poor study which did not define the intervention. In planning your own evaluation you will need to specify clearly the programme or change which you are to evaluate before you can start. The diagram forces you to think about what is 'in the box' and what is not.

The diagram also shows any before-and-after measures and when they were made, the timescale and the number of people involved. In the rehabilitation example there were three sets of measures before and after: sick leave, self-reports of pain and mobility and functioning. The diagram would show 61 patients going into the active rehabilitation 'box' and 53 remaining at two years, and 46 going into the traditional rehabilitation 'box' and 40 remaining at two years. Appendix 2 shows the box diagram drawing for this example evaluation.

The next chapters use this basic diagram to show the six most common types of evaluation design in healthcare. When looking through these, consider which diagram best represents the design which the evaluators used in the rehabilitation example. There is no single best design, only the design which is feasible within the evaluation constraints and most suited to the purposes of the evaluation, which is to answer the users' questions and help them to make more informed decisions. The next chapters will help you to choose the right design for your evaluation.

Box 7.1: Drawing a design for an evaluation

- Describe the intervention, targets and outcome.
- Use the box diagram to draw the design.
- In the box, describe the intervention and show the measures and when they were implemented.

- Note any key features of the environment 'surrounding' the box.
- Show the targets (how many?) and note characteristics about the target on which you will need to gather data.
- Note possible confounders and what controls were made.
- Note other explanations for outcomes, apart from the intervention.
- Draw all this on one side of A4 paper.

Overview of the six designs

There are six main designs used for health evaluations and these are described in the next two chapters.

1 *Descriptive* (type 1): a description of features of the programme, policy or implementation process.
2 *Audit* (type 2): a comparison of what is done with specified standards or objectives.
3 *Outcome* (type 3): the 'before' state of targets of the intervention compared to their 'after' or 'later' state.
4 *Comparative* (type 4): a comparison of the before-and-after states of people who received two or more different interventions.
5 *Randomised controlled trial* (RCT) (type 5): a comparison of a specified before-and-after state of people who were randomly allocated to an intervention or to a placebo or a comparison intervention.
6 *Intentional change to organisation* (type 6) which looks at an intervention to an organisation or to health providers and at the before-and-after effects of the intervention on these targets (type 6a) or on patients (type 6b).

Apart from type 5, all designs can be used prospectively or retrospectively. Most concurrent designs use type 1 and 2, although some concurrent evaluations are made over a sufficiently long period to be able to gather data about outcomes. Different designs answer different questions and, in general, type 6 and 5 designs are more expensive and take longer than type 4 which costs more than type 3, and so on. Whether the extra time and cost are worth it depends on for whom we are doing the evaluation and their questions. An evaluation does not need to be a type 5 experimental RCT or type 4 comparative design to be useful: it depends on who the evaluation is for, their questions and their criteria of valuation. An RCT may be too expensive and take too long for some users or may not be practical or may be unethical. Evaluations are to help people make better informed decisions than they would otherwise do. However, a poorly designed and conducted evaluation is worse than none at all because it may be misleading.

The 'NIPOO' model

We finish this chapter by noting a useful model which helps to separate the different subjects of a programme or change evaluation and indicate which data to collect. This is the Needs-Input-Process-Output-Outcome (NIPOO) model.

Box 7.2: The NIPOO model of a programme change

Environment

Needs → Inputs → Processes → Outputs → Outcome

Targets   For targets

                                           For others

                                           Short term and long term

---

The 'environment' is the many factors surrounding the intervention process which may affect the outcomes. For health programmes, 'needs' refers to the health needs of the targets who receive the intervention. In the rehabilitation example, the targets are people suffering from neck and shoulder disorders and their main health needs are for cure or symptom relief. 'Inputs' refers to all that 'goes into' the intervention. The evaluation will select which inputs to describe according to the evaluation users' needs for information. This may include a description of the intervention resources (e.g. the number and type of personnel working in the programme and the amount of time they give) and of the targets (e.g. the number and characteristics of the patients). In our example there was no description of resources for either programme, but there was a description of 'input' patient characteristics.

The 'process' is how the intervention is carried out and describes the different components, activities and procedures performed. There was little description of the process for either the active or traditional rehabilitation in the example evaluation report. 'Outputs' are the immediate products of the process and are often described in terms of the number of patients who complete the process: in our example we do not know how many patients finished each programme, only the numbers at two years for the follow-up data collection. 'Outcomes' are the difference the programme makes to the target patients and to others, in both the short and long term. In the example differences were measured before and at two years for sick leave, pain and mobility and functioning for the target patients. No other outcomes were measured or reported.

The NIPOO model also demonstrates how value criteria which are often used in programme evaluations can be measured. Efficiency is the ratio of inputs to outputs for one programme compared to another. For example, if the resource inputs for treating 50 patients with the active rehabilitation is costed at $25 000, then the cost per patient is $500. Efficiency is only really meaningful when compared with another programme, so we would also calculate the input-output ratio for the traditional programme. This may turn out to be $350 per patient, which would make the traditional programme more efficient.

But is the traditional programme more effective? In the example we compare measures before and after to find the outcomes and we discover that the outcomes are similar for the active and traditional programmes. Here we are defining effectiveness as whether the programme meets the health needs of people for whom it is intended. To describe effectiveness we compare the health needs of people before with their needs after. Note, however, that there are other ways of defining efficiency and effectiveness; effectiveness is sometimes viewed as whether the programme met its objectives, even if meeting needs was not an objective.

Summary

- Evaluation is a service to a user and the best evaluation design is the one which best meets their needs within the constraints of the study.
- To understand an evaluation it is necessary to identify which type of design was used. The basis for planning an evaluation is deciding which design to use.
- An evaluation can be retrospective, looking backwards at what happened, or prospective, looking forwards at what might happen, or concurrent, looking at what is happening now.
- An evaluation design is a model of the key features of an evaluation. It shows in a note form the intervention, targets, timescale and data collected.

- To understand an evaluation report and to decide on a design, it helps to draw a diagram with:
  - a 'box' around what was evaluated (the intervention)
  - any before-and-after measures and when they were implemented
  - the timescale and the number of people involved.
- There are six main types of design:
  - type 1: descriptive (some action evaluations, case study evaluations)
  - type 2: audit (comparing what is done with standards or with the objectives of the intervention)
  - type 3: before-and-after
  - type 4: comparative before-and-after
  - type 5: randomised controlled trial
  - type 6: intentional change to organisation(s), (6a) effects on providers or (6b) effects on patients/population of intervention to providers.
- The Needs-Input-Process-Outputs-Outcomes (NIPOO) model helps to separate the different subjects of an evaluation and to see which data are needed or are missing.

Chapter 8

Process evaluation designs

Introduction

Before looking at whether a health programme or change is effective, we may need to describe exactly what it is and which people have received it. Process evaluations are undertaken to discover how a programme or change is implemented and whether it is being implemented as planned. They do not look at outcomes, but may look at whether the people for whom the intervention is intended do in fact get it. Process evaluations usually look at whether the intervention is carried out in accordance with standards, procedures or objectives. They can be made prospectively, but usually they are retrospective or concurrent.

Some 'audits' which do not look at outcomes are examples of process evaluations, as are most action evaluations which give fast feedback to decision makers about a programme or change. This chapter describes two designs for a process evaluation: descriptive and audit. These are used where it is not possible to collect outcome data for reasons of cost or time. They may also be used when people are not clear about exactly what they want evaluated or whether an intervention has actually been implemented.

Type 1: descriptive

If a descriptive type 1 design had been used to evaluate the rehabilitation programme described in Chapter 6, then the evaluators would have simply described the active and the traditional programmes – the different activities which the programmes carried out and how they were organised. The evaluator does not just observe and describe, but is influenced by concepts and theories to decide what to describe and how to conceptualise the intervention: there is usually a theoretical framework to guide the description. These designs can also describe strengths and weaknesses of the programmes as perceived by those interviewed.

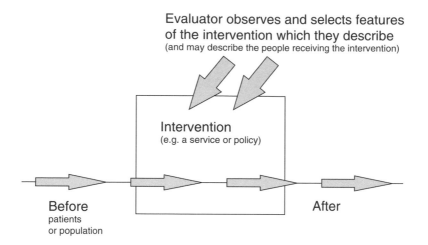

Figure 8.1 Descriptive evalaution design.

Although there are no data about outcomes, peoples' expectations can be reported, making this a quick way to do a simple evaluation.

The description would probably note features of the context or 'host organisation' which helped or hindered setting up and running the programme (the 'intervention context' or 'environment'). Such features might include whether the rehabilitation unit had a history of successful teamwork and any changes which were introduced to the programme over time, for example if there were significant personnel changes.

A descriptive design might also be appropriate to describe a change which is thought to have had an impact on employees' health, but where there is some uncertainty as to exactly what was changed. In this case the change is considered an intervention and the descriptive design is used just to get a good description of what the change was.

The purpose of this evaluation design is to describe the intervention and 'important' features of the 'environment' surrounding the intervention. The design does not measure outcomes and some would say it is not a 'real evaluation' design but a descriptive or case study research design. The typical questions answered by this design are: what is it and what was or is being done?

Sometimes a descriptive evaluation is needed by managers who are remote from what is happening. After discussion, the evaluator may find that managers do not have the time or money for an outcome evaluation and actually only want a description of 'what is really happening' by an independent observer. Another reason to do a descriptive evaluation of an existing programme or policy is to give a precise description which allows other people to set up a similar programme or to carry out a similar policy. Also, it may be premature to try to judge the value of something if there is not an agreed and explicit description of it as implemented, which is the case with many health reforms or policies. Good descriptive evaluations make hypotheses about possible outcomes and about possible causes of and hindrances to outcomes. They can generate theory about the intervention and how it works which can be further tested using other methods. This is important when assessing changes or programmes which are being rapidly developed.

The strengths of this type of design are that it does not need many resources, can be done in collaboration with service providers and people receiving a treatment and can clarify objectives and highlight problems. Its weaknesses are that it can be ignored as unscientific, biased or trivial and does not give data about the effects. The usefulness of such evaluations depends on the skill, knowledge and credibility of the evaluator and the theoretical perspective which they use to select and conceptualise what to describe – a descriptive evaluation by a health economist would be different from one done by an anthropologist or psychologist.

Some would say that we cannot really call a simple description like the type 1 design an evaluation. But sometimes evaluation users are not exactly sure what 'it' is that they want to evaluate, what 'its' aims are or what questions they want answered (i.e. they are unsure about what is 'in the box'). Evaluators can be too quick to propose a sophisticated and expensive design when more consideration of the user's concerns and questions would show that all they need is an independent description, which then helps them to judge value or plan another type of evaluation.

Descriptive evaluations can be used to describe a new or unfamiliar health programme or policy, but are more often used to describe a service or policy which is unclear or which is in the early stages of evolution. Descriptive evaluations may or may not describe the costs of an intervention. They can be prospective but most are retrospective (e.g. many 'summative' evaluations) or concurrent (e.g. many 'developmental', 'action' or 'formative' evaluations).

If the description uses explicit standards and criteria to decide what to describe or to compare the programme against, then it is a type 2 audit design. If the description involves a before–after comparison, then it is a type 3 outcome evaluation (*see* Chapter 9).

Type 2: audit

An audit design for the rehabilitation example would require a description of procedures and standards for the rehabilitation programme. The

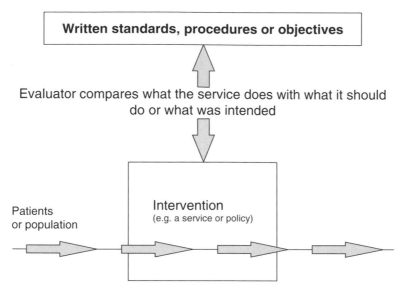

Figure 8.2 Audit evaluation design.

evaluation would then compare these to what the programme personnel actually did, using documentation, observation and interviews. This is what many 'quality assurance' or 'compliance' evaluations do. This may be an appropriate design if users wanted to know if the programme was implemented according to specification.

Another variety of this design would be to compare the programme with the statement of objectives and assess the extent to which these were met (sometimes called 'effectiveness evaluation'). One objective may be to ensure that all the people in need of the programme do in fact receive it or that it is equitably provided. This then could be used as a standard against which the programme is evaluated. If there are objectives in terms of outcomes, such as curing or reducing patient symptoms, then a type 3 design would be required which is discussed in the next chapter.

The question this design answers is, did the intervention follow procedures or achieve the objectives and/or standards set for it? The purpose of the design is to judge the value of what people are doing by comparing what they do with what they are supposed to do. The design is used for: inspection, compliance monitoring, managerial monitoring of policy implementation, simple economic audits, developmental self or peer review exercises and some types of quality assurance and clinical audit.

This design is like a type 1 descriptive evaluation, but it describes the health intervention or policy in comparison with intended objectives, procedures, standards or norms which are usually specified in writing.

The audit may be carried out by external evaluators or by the organisation itself using established standards. The weaknesses of the design are that it depends on having a clearly specified set of standards, procedures or objectives (e.g. a clear law or statement of policy) or on creating such a set as part of the evaluation. However, these are often not clear, for example, there may be no implementation plan against which to compare what people are doing.

The design does not help to judge the value of the intervention, but just whether people 'follow orders'; there is an assumption that if people follow procedures then they are doing something of value. This may be valid, for example where it is already known that the intervention is effective and the procedures describe exactly what people should do to get the results, e.g. an 'evidence-based' intervention. However, the intervention itself may be ineffective or inappropriate. The strengths of the design are that few resources are needed, it can be done quickly and it is good for self-evaluation. It can help to explain why a policy or intervention fails or succeeds and can sometimes yield knowledge which can be generalised.

Audit designs assume that if the service providers followed the standards then a beneficial outcome will follow, but this may not have been proven before. This evaluation design does not discover effects or possible causes, but it can be used to audit outcome or performance, for example how well an employer complies with employee rights or safety standards. Checking whether practitioners are following treatment guidelines is one type of audit evaluation. However, the term 'clinical audit' also describes clinicians first deciding which guidelines and criteria to use: if this decision is based on evidence of effectiveness, then the audit has more value. Other types of audit evaluations are of services, for example a quality assurance audit of a health service using a set of quality standards, or a policy audit to check whether people are complying with a policy. Audits are usually retrospective or concurrent and may or may not consider costs.

Some would not consider audits to be a type of evaluation: the design does not aim to evaluate the effectiveness of the intervention but whether people carry out procedures or achieve objectives or meet standards. 'Monitoring' is a better term to describe many of the activities which use this design, but we are here taking a broad view of evaluation and include audits as one form of evaluation. One reason for so doing is because information about whether people or services meet specifications or objectives is increasingly necessary to judge the value of what they are doing, where specifications and objectives are based on evidence about what is effective. Generally the value of audits depends on the validity of the guidelines, standards, procedures or objectives and whether these are evidence-based and derived from evaluations carried out using other designs.

Summary

- Process evaluations are carried out when people want to know how a programme or change is implemented, whether it is implemented as planned or meets specifications or are uncertain about what exactly the intervention is which is to be evaluated.
- The two designs used for process evaluations are the descriptive (type 1) and the audit (type 2) designs.
- The disadvantage of the descriptive (type 1) design is that it does not give data about the results of the intervention but it can report peoples' expectations and their assessments of the strengths and weaknesses of the intervention.
- The advantages are that it is less costly than other designs and is useful for describing complex interventions or changes such as a health reform or a programme which has not been tried before. The value of the description for the user depends on the skills and theoretical perspective of the evaluator, which affect what the evaluator 'sees' and describes.
- The advantages of the audit (type 2) design are that it is not expensive and can be done quickly, if the standards and procedures are well described. It is useful for evaluating interventions which are known to be effective and where evaluation users want to assess whether people are following procedures and achieving standards for compliance evaluations or quality assurance.
- The disadvantages of the audit design are that it does not give data about outcomes and there is a risk that the standards may not be appropriate for the local setting or based on the latest research.
- An evaluation can use one or more designs. Some outcome evaluations can also use these type 1 or 2 process designs to help understand how the intervention produces the outcome, for example by building an EITO model to understand the environment-intervention-target-outcome pattern (*see* Box 6.3).

Chapter 9

Outcome evaluation designs

Introduction

Outcome evaluations designs aim to find out the effects of an intervention. These designs answer the question 'Does it work?' or 'Does it work better than the alternative?' They do this by comparing the target people or organisations before and after the intervention; for example, by comparing patients' states before and after receiving a service or by comparing the health of a population before and after a health programme or change is introduced. Some may also try to find out if the intervention makes a difference to people other than the targets. For example, what effect does it have on health personnel or patients' carers? The type 6 designs use the before-and-after design to look at the effects of an intervention to an organisation, such as a training programme or a health reform.

Some designs do not measure before and after but just ask people retrospectively if they thought the intervention had an effect. The difference between the designs is in the degree of certainty which each gives about whether the outcomes were actually produced by the intervention.

Type 3: single before-and-after

If this design was used in the rehabilitation example in Box 6.1, the evaluation would only have looked at the active rehabilitation service and would not also have looked at the outcomes for the traditional service. It would have been less expensive to do so, but we would not know if the outcomes were better or worse than the usual service which people received in primary care.

The box drawing shows that people 'pass through' an intervention and are then no longer exposed to it. The drawing thus can be misleading for some types of interventions which do not stop working on patients or for many health reforms or polices. Sometimes people continue receiving the service – the 'box' is not closed on the right side. Examples are

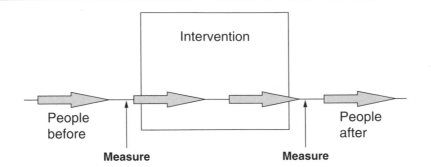

Figure 9.1: Type 3: single before-and-after.

medication for hypertension, interventions for chronic disorders or home care services. For these, the diagram shows that a measure is taken before they start and then at periods after first receiving the treatment.

This is the simplest type of design for discovering if an intervention may have made a difference to the people receiving it. It is often designed as an experiment and the evaluator predicts the effects of the intervention on the targets. It can be used retrospectively where the evaluator looks back at before-and-after states. The purpose of the design is to help to judge the value of an intervention by comparing the state of people or organisations before with their state after the intervention using outcome data or measures. The questions this design aims to answer are: what are the effects or what difference does the intervention make to the target?

The before–after comparison may be of one specific feature of the people before and after (e.g. blood pressure, stress levels or how many attend the clinic in a month) or of a number of features (e.g. a set of employee perceptions, physical measures, providers' assessments of 'patient progress', employee income losses, etc.). The before–after comparisons are based on theories and predictions about the possible effects of the intervention.

The weakness of the design is that it cannot give conclusive evidence of effects. This is because, if a before–after difference is found, it may have been caused by things other than the intervention. The difference may be due to selecting subjects who would show these effects over time anyway; for example, patients' health state would have improved without the intervention. The many possible confounding variables are not controlled, controls being one way to exclude variables as explanations for the effects.

The strength is that evaluations using this design can be small scale and relatively quick. The design can use few resources if the evaluator selects a small number of subjects, makes one or a few simple before-and-after measures and makes the measurement soon after the intervention. This makes it a useful design for practical professional self-evaluation or in a quality project.

Compared to the process designs 1 and 2 described in the last chapter, this design is, for many, the first recognisable evaluation design because it looks at outcome. However, those who take this view would also be dissatisfied with how this design tries to discover the effect of the intervention: how does this design prove that the difference is due to the intervention and not to something else? Would the difference have happened anyway without an intervention?

One way to improve this design is to gather a series of 'before' data and a series of 'after' data rather than just gathering data once 'before' and once 'after'. For example, a simple type 3 design might gather 'time series' data about how many people attend a clinic over one month before and one month after an intervention which publicises the clinic. An improved type 3 design could gather data about monthly attendance for each of three months before and three months after the intervention. By doing this we can see the variability of attendance over time which will happen for many reasons and then get a better idea whether the difference before and after the intervention is significant. Another way is a time series design which stops the intervention and starts it again and studies whether the targets revert to their 'before' states after the intervention is stopped and then show changes when the intervention is started again.

Type 4: comparative

The questions addressed by this design are: what are the effects of the intervention, compared to a similar intervention or to the status quo elsewhere? The rehabilitation example used a design of this type: it compared the before-and-after measures for two groups, one of which received the active rehabilitation and the other the traditional rehabilitation. The design is also used, for example, for economic evaluations of two different employment policies or an evaluation of a health reform or policy in one area compared to the status quo elsewhere. It could be used to evaluate a training programme compared to a written information intervention or to compare two or more different types of services.

The design is like a type 3 outcome evaluation, but compares the outcomes of two groups undergoing different interventions. Normally it is carried out prospectively, but retrospective type 4 designs are possible (e.g. some comparative evaluations of different policies or working

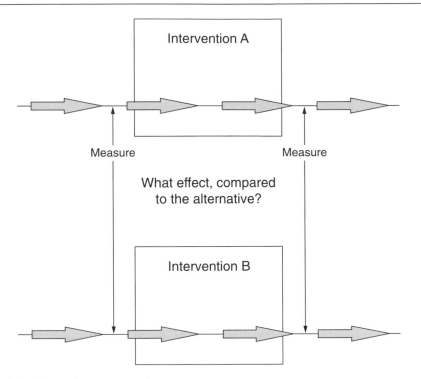

Figure 9.2: Type 4: comparative.

conditions). One variation of the design is a comparison of end-states only, rather than a comparison of the before–after change (outcome).

The weaknesses of the design are that it is expensive and difficult to prove that the effects were due to the interventions alone, rather than due to other factors. The strengths are that, if the design is made with care, such evaluations can suggest which of the two interventions is more effective or cost-effective. The design is suitable where it is unethical or impractical to treat or intervene with only one group.

Unlike type 3 designs, this design compares two interventions. It is a common design for evaluations of services or health programmes, for example where a new service is started at one site which people want to compare with a traditional service at another site. An example is a comparison of the health state of patients before and after a new service for stroke patients compared to conventional rehabilitation. Evaluations with these designs are often carried out according to experimental principles ('controlled trials'), with hypotheses to test and with different methods for controlling for influences other than the interventions, such as patient characteristics (e.g. age, sex, severity of illness, duration of previous illness, etc.). A common control technique is 'matching' the characteristics of the people experiencing each intervention, which was done in the example evaluation. The aim of matching is to try to exclude influences other than the intervention which might affect the outcome, but matching is less good for this purpose than random allocation (see design 5 below). Typical matching criteria for patients are age, sex and socio-economic status.

The design, like the type 3 design, can also be used when conditions allow a 'natural experiment'. An example is to make a retrospective evaluation where there are records or measures already available. Comparative outcome evaluations of this type can give some objective evidence of the effect of one intervention compared to another but they take longer and use more resources than type 3 designs. The cost and time required increase with more subjects (which calls for more time and care matching subjects), with more complex measures (e.g. quality of life measures), with more than one 'after' measure and with measurement some time after the intervention.

The difference between the type 4 and type 3 designs is that two interventions are compared and the difference between type 4 and type 5 is that people are not randomly allocated. Also in type 4, one of the interventions is not a placebo: the controls are therefore fewer than for a type 5 full experimental design which uses a placebo.

Type 5: randomised controlled trial

This design is not suitable for evaluations of most types of health programme, policy or reforms. It is included here to show the design which is best known and respected in medical research and is the standard against which many other designs are judged in healthcare, often inappropriately.

The idea behind this design is to create two groups which are exactly the same in all respects apart from the fact that one (target) group received the intervention. The design can rule out many alternative explanations for a change which is detected in the targets and can give evidence of causal mechanisms. The design answers the question: what are the effects of the intervention, compared to a control group? It is used for an experimental and economic evaluation to gain evidence of the probable effect of a treatment or service on one or a few measures of the health state of a group of patients.

This design is the 'classic' evaluation design which many think of as the 'proper' evaluation for a treatment or a service. It is like the type 4 design, but the people selected for the intervention are randomly

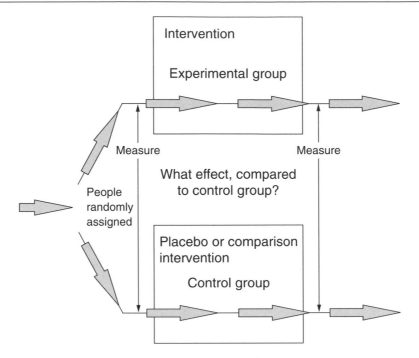

Figure 9.3: Type 5: randomised controlled trial.

assigned to a control (sometimes a placebo) and an intervention group. This allows statistical methods to be used to compare the outcomes and assess if the difference between the groups is greater than would be expected by chance alone. Using statistics we can predict that by chance alone anything up to 5% of people may show an effect of the intervention. We want to be sure that the difference in effect is significantly greater than what we would expect by chance. This requires not only randomisation but a large enough number of subjects to be entered into the experiment to be sure that any differences are statistically significant.

The design is able to reduce the number of possible explanations for any differences between the outcomes for the two groups being due to patient characteristics. Ideally the second control group do not 'get nothing' but receive an intervention called a 'placebo' which is as similar as possible but without the 'active ingredient' (one estimate is that 30–40% of patients will show an improvement without any intervention). Also subjects do not know which group they are in (the subjects are 'blind') and the service providers do not know who is in which group (provider blinding). Such double blinding is not always possible.

The weaknesses of the design are that it is expensive, takes time, needs many carefully selected patients and evaluators with experience, skill and statistical expertise to produce credible results. Often these designs do not examine patients' subjective experiences and may lose important effects for a few individuals in the group average. The design has been criticised as not allowing generalisation of findings to normal settings because the subjects are carefully selected (to maximise controls) which means that the subjects are not typical of those in normal settings; the design maximises 'internal' validity at the expense of 'external' validity. Nine other criticisms are listed in Øvretveit (1998a).

The strength is that the design gives more reliable and valid information about the effect of the intervention than type 3 simple outcome evaluation or a type 4 non-random, non-placebo comparison. The results from a well-conducted evaluation using this design have high credibility with most clinicians. In principle the design can be retrospective but, when looking back over time, it is usually difficult to get true randomisation or a good control group or to check if the intervention was stable. Type 5 designs are prospective and called 'experimental' because the evaluator intervenes to create a change and then studies it using similar principles and controls to those used by a natural scientist in a laboratory. Note, however, that whilst randomisation gives control over patient characteristics, control is also needed over the interventions to keep them constant and subject to the same environmental influences, and this is more difficult.

Some of the principles can be applied in programme or reform evaluations, such as randomly assigning providers or units rather than patients to an intervention and a control group. But this may not be possible and 'blinding' of subjects may be very difficult. The full design is not suitable for evaluating many health interventions because of the difficulties of controlling for extraneous variables or of controlling the intervention itself. However, for some interventions, such as many diagnostic or treatment interventions, there is no doubt that it can be the best design for answering certain questions, if the resources and time are available.

> *People criticise the randomised controlled trial. But if I had cancer and did not know which treatment to take, or whether to take any, it is only evidence from such trials that I would use to make my decisions. I would not stake my life on evidence from less powerful designs.*
>
> *If I had cancer and had to choose a treatment I would want to know what the treatment experience is like and what other patients thought about the treatment process. There is no point in living for five years more if the treatment is so awful you cannot live properly.*

Which view do you hold?

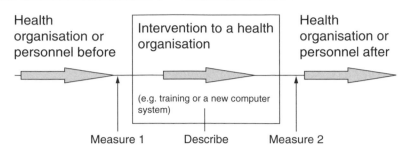

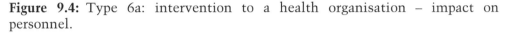

Figure 9.4: Type 6a: intervention to a health organisation – impact on personnel.

Type 6a: intervention to a health organisation – impact on personnel

The two type 6 designs consider the effect of an intervention on a health organisation. Examples are evaluations of a training programme for physicians, an intranet system, a new nursing protocol or a new financing system. The type 6a design answers the question: 'What is the effect of an intervention to a service on health personnel or organisation?' It is similar to the before–after type 3 design. The purpose of this design is to judge the value of an intervention to a service by comparing the state of health personnel or organisational functioning before and after the intervention.

The data to be gathered before and after depend on the user's questions and future decisions, the objectives of the intervention and any theories about how the intervention may affect personnel or organisation. Common methods are surveys, observation and measures such as personnel work stress. Before-and-after data could also be about resources, as in an economic evaluation of the effect of an intervention, such as new technology, on the service costs.

The weakness is, as with type 3, that it is difficult to be sure that any effects on health personnel or organisational functioning detected are only due to the intervention and not to other influences. One variation of this design is to use a comparison organisation to control for some factors. Another weakness for some purposes is that it does not consider the effect on patients; if a change to health personnel or organisation is detected, how does this change affect patients? The strengths are that it is cheap, quick and usually better than nothing, so long as the limitations are spelled out. It is more useful when another evaluation has already discovered how the intervention or its outcome for providers affects patient care.

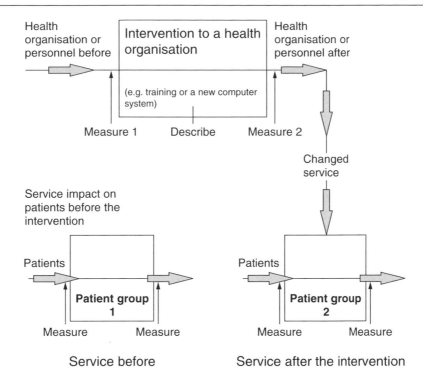

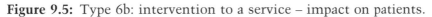

Figure 9.5: Type 6b: intervention to a service – impact on patients.

Type 6b: intervention to a service – impact on patients

This design looks at the effect of an intervention to organisation on patients, as well as the effect on health personnel or organisational functioning. By comparing patient outcomes before and after the change, the design can help to judge the value of a change to organisation or of other interventions to a service. It is used for evaluations of training programmes, quality assurance and other interventions intended to improve patient care.

The two patient groups studied before and after the intervention to organisation is made need to be carefully matched to increase certainty that any difference in outcome between them is due to the intervention and not to the characteristics of the patients. Variations of this design involve comparing two or more services receiving the intervention and the effects on the patients of these services.

The weakness of this design is that it is difficult to match or control for patient characteristics between the before-and-after groups. Also the measures chosen to study the effect of the service on patients might not detect important benefits or disbenefits produced by the intervention. Its strength is that it does give a method for assessing how changes to health organisations affect patient care, whether or not this is the primary aim of the change or intervention. This design and variations of it allow an evaluation of the impact on patients and on health personnel.

Summary

- Outcome evaluation designs are used to find out if an intervention or action has any effects. The design measures the state of target people or organisations before and after the intervention to see if it makes a difference.
- The simple before–after type 3 design is low cost and easy to arrange, but it cannot give conclusive evidence of effects. If a before–after difference is found, we cannot be sure if the difference was caused by things other than the intervention.
- The comparative type 4 design compares the before–after difference in two groups of people or organisations, one of which receives the test intervention and the other receives a traditional or comparable intervention. If both groups are similar and both interventions take place in a similar environment, then it is likely that any difference in the before–after states of the groups is due to the interventions alone.
- The randomised controlled trial type 5 design allocates patients or other subjects randomly to the test intervention and to a comparison intervention or a placebo, which is the same as the test but without the active ingredient. Any difference between the two groups which is greater than chance is significant if confounders are controlled for.
- The type 6a design is used to evaluate the effect of an intervention such as a training programme or health reform on health providers or organisational functioning. The type 6b design is used when the effects of such interventions on patients or populations are also of interest.

Chapter 10

Assessing an evaluation and choosing a design

Introduction

Should we act on the findings of this evaluation report? This is a question frequently faced by health personnel, politicians and their advisors. The ability to assess an evaluation quickly is a skill which we all need. The problem is that there are so many different types of evaluation and it seems that we need to be experts to make a proper assessment. However, for most purposes it is possible quickly to assess most types of evaluation by answering the simple questions given in the assessment guide in the first part of this chapter.

Assessing others' evaluations is good practice for designing our own evaluation: we see the mistakes they make and what we need to consider in our own design. Which design to use in our evaluation is a question evaluators should consider, even if the answer seems obvious: looking at the alternatives helps to point out the strengths and weaknesses of our chosen design. The second part of this chapter gives guidelines for defining the most important features of an evaluation and for using this to decide the best design for your circumstances. Choosing the design is one step in planning an evaluation – details of planning are discussed in Part 1 of the book.

After reading this chapter you should be able to:

- quickly but systematically assess any evaluation report
- work through a method to decide which design to use in an evaluation and use this to plan an evaluation.

How to assess an evaluation: the '4D' method

The previous chapters gave the tools to understand an evaluation by working out what was the intervention, the target and the outcome findings and described the challenge which evaluators face when they have to prove that the outcome was caused by the intervention and not by something else. We saw how evaluation design can control for confounders or, where we cannot control, how we can use multiple data sources and other methods to assess the effect which confounders might have on the outcome.

But understanding an evaluation is not sufficient to decide the implications for our work or organisation. We need to do more than analyse an evaluation and represent it in a diagram. Practitioners, managers and policy makers need to be able to assess the quality of an evaluation and its relevance to their situation to help them decide what action to take. There is guidance for assessing medical research evaluations of treatments (Crombie, 1996; Greenhalgh, 1997), but these methods are often not appropriate for assessing evaluations of health programmes, policies or changes and other types of evaluation in healthcare (Hawe *et al.*, 1990; Heron, 1986; Scott and Weston, 1998). Other frameworks have been developed for assessing health economic evaluations (Drummond *et al.*, 1987), and evaluations of educational interventions (EGGE, 1999).

The '4D' method can be used for assessing any type of evaluation. This method asks four sets of questions about:

1 the way the report describes the intervention
2 the quality of the data
3 whether the design excludes other possible explanations for the findings
4 the relevance of the findings to your work or to the evaluation user's questions.

1 Description

The first assessment is of how well the report describes the intervention. For the example rehabilitation evaluation in Box 6.1, what score would you give the description in the report of both the multidisciplinary and the traditional primary care rehabilitation interventions? (0 is very poor and 5 is excellent.) Have the evaluators described the different components of the intervention (for example, any education given to the patients, the type of assessment the patients received)? Are any changes to the intervention described (is it constant)? One test of a good description is: could we repeat the intervention and be confident of getting the same results?

2   Data

The second assessment looks first at the data gathered about outcomes. In the rehabilitation example, would you score the quality of data-gathering and analysis as 4: very good? Your score depends on whether you think the measures are valid and reliable. Also, do the measures relate to value criteria which are important to the evaluation users? When and how often were they collected? If the data consist of stakeholders' perceptions when they look backwards at the effects, then were these perceptions gathered in a way which properly used the methods described in Chapter 11 and was triangulation used?

So far the data assessment only refers to how well the evaluators used the data-gathering methods and analysis. But there may be outcome data which you think were missing, for example patient satisfaction with the services. Note this because it helps later when thinking about the relevance of this evaluation for your work or organisation. Are there data missing about the resources used (costs)?

The second data assessment is to look at other data presented about the targets (e.g. patient's age) and about the environment (e.g. were the services private or public?). Which data were gathered about these subjects and how reliable and valid are these data? Reliability refers to whether someone else would find the same things if they used the same methods. Validity here refers to whether the right methods were used to gather data about the variables that were studied, for example socio-economic status. It also refers to whether other data should have been gathered about features of the targets and the environment, for example the level of unemployment in the area.

The purpose of this data assessment is to look at how well the data were gathered and if there are any data missing about features of the targets and environment which are important to understanding what caused the outcomes. The example evaluation in Chapter 6 collected enough data about changes in people's work task and the workplace to be able to report that these changes seemed to have more impact on outcomes than the interventions, but no more details were given.

3   Design

The third assessment is whether anything else could explain the findings. Are all confounders considered? Which are controlled for? Which are not excluded from possible influence on the targets? Did the design introduce factors which would bias the results in favour of the intervention or against it? For example, in a type 4 comparison study, were the target people or organisations sufficiently similar to be sure that differences in outcome were due to the intervention alone?

We saw in the last chapter that the rehabilitation example used the type 4 comparative design. As both the rehabilitation programmes were carried out in the same geographical area, this gave a control for some environmental influences. But it was not possible to control for changes in the workplace which could affect the outcome measures. The evaluators comment that changes in work task and workplace had more effect than the intervention, but the design did not collect enough data about this to draw conclusions. Does this mean that you would give the design a low score: 2 rather than 4 or 5?

4   Decision relevance

There are two ways of assessing decision relevance: in terms of whether the findings are relevant and useful to the evaluation users or in terms of whether they are relevant to your work and organisation.

Are the conclusions justified by the evidence presented? This is the first question to ask when assessing the decision relevance. If they are not then the findings are not useful to the users or to you. Another general question asked by editors of journals when reviewing evaluations is: could anything reported mislead an average reader and what might be the consequences?

In the rehabilitation example, is the conclusion that there is no difference between the multidisciplinary and traditional rehabilitation justified by the evidence? We can conclude that the outcomes which were measured are similar for the two programmes because the report gives enough details of the targets, the outcomes and data-gathering methods to justify this conclusion. But do we know enough about the confounders to be sure that these outcomes were only due to the programmes? Also, are there other outcomes which may be more important but which were not measured, such as the cost of each programme per patient?

Can the findings be generalised to the user's situation or to your situation? This is the second decision relevance question. We may conclude that the conclusions are justified, but that the programmes in Sweden are not similar to our rehabilitation programmes. For example, our primary healthcare programme may be multidisciplinary and 'active'. There may also be environmental differences: for example, the amount of money paid for sick leave. The question is: what is different in the evaluation from your (or the user's) situation and does this mean that the findings have no relevance to your decisions (or to the users')?

Applying your assessment

To make your assessment specific it is useful to give a score for each of the above '4Ds'. The following shows how one group of managers in a workshop on evaluation scored the rehabilitation example, using the '4D' assessment method.

> *Description: score 2.*
> *Poor description of the two rehabilitation programmes. The main components of the multidisciplinary programme were described but in not enough detail. Little was said about the traditional programme. We could not see exactly what the differences were between the two types of programme. We could not reconstruct the programme in our area from the description given.*

> *Data: score 3*
> *The measures used before and after to gather data about the patients did relate to the value criteria which are important to managers and professionals. The methods for gathering data about sick leave, symptoms and functional ability are validated. As far as we can tell the methods were applied correctly in the study. There were no data about cost outcomes. Enough data was given about targets and the environment around the programmes to judge possible confounders.*

> *Design: score 4*
> *This was a good design for answering the users' questions. Managers and occupational health professionals want to know the difference between work-based programmes of this type and traditional primary care, and so a type 4 comparison was the right one. There was also a reasonably long-term follow-up of two years.*

> *Decision relevance: score 3*
> *For managers and professionals in Sweden, the findings could help to make more informed decisions about whether to set up a work-based rehabilitation programme of this type or even whether to change the organisation of a traditional primary care programme. We do not think the findings could be generalised elsewhere.*

Box 10.1: The '4D' assessment method for an evaluation study (score 0–5 for each)

1 *Description?*
Is the action, change or 'intervention' well described? (The components? Are any changes in the intervention described? Is intervention separated from other change/things? Do you know enough from the description to repeat it?)

2 *Data?*
Are the measures or other types of data collected about outcomes or targets true or an artifact of the researcher or method? (Valid? Reliable? When? How long for? How often? Sample?) Are there outcomes which are more important to the user of the evaluation that were not collected?

3 *Design?*
Could anything else explain the findings? (Are all confounders considered? Which are controlled for? Does the design exclude other explanations? Were these predicted at the start of the study? Does the analysis consider and account for other explanations?).

4 *Decision relevance?*
How relevant is the study for your situation and the action/change you are considering? (What is similar to and different from your situation in terms of the action, the target and the context?)

How to choose a design

The next part of this chapter gives guidance for choosing a design, bearing in mind how others will assess the evaluation which you carry out. The best practice for designing an evaluation is critically to assess other evaluation studies, using an assessment method such as the '4D' method described above. The following gives guidance for choosing a design by asking eight questions which show which types of design you might use and illustrating this with the rehabilitation evaluation example. These questions ask you to think about features of the intervention you are evaluating, its environment and the targets of the intervention.

1   How controllable are the intervention and confounders?

How specific and stable is the intervention? In the example, the evaluators could control the rehabilitation programmes to some degree over the eight weeks so that the programmes were similar for each patient and were constant. But how controllable were other confounders such as features of the target and of the environment? It was possible to control for some confounders such as patient characteristics by selecting patients. The evaluators were able to exclude those with neck and shoulder disorders caused by trauma, rheumatic diseases or pregnancy. It was also possible to control for some environmental confounders if they used a comparison programme in the same area, such as a traditional primary care programme.

2   Can you describe and specify the intervention? (If not, then a type 1 descriptive design is necessary)

This question follows on from the first because a controllable intervention is usually one which can be specified and described. In the example, both interventions could be well described, even though the report did not give a good description.

If the answer had been that it was difficult to describe and control the intervention then a type 1 descriptive design would be needed, possibly followed by another design in a phase 2 evaluation.

3   Can you compare the intentions of the programme or reform to what was done? Are objectives or procedures specified? (If so, a type 2 design is possible)

This could have been done in the example because some objectives were stated for the rehabilitation programme and some procedures and standards were specified; a type 2 audit design was feasible. But this would not have answered the users' questions; their value criteria were not whether the programme met objectives or standards but whether patients were better able to work, had less pain and could take up previous activities.

4 Can you compare targets before and after the intervention? (type 3)

Meaningful before-and-after measures of the targets could be made in the example evaluation. There were standard measures available and these could be used, making a type 3 design one option to consider. But would this answer the users' questions? Would they be sure that any before–after differences were caused by the rehabilitation programme and not something else?

5 Can you compare the intervention to a comparison? (nothing or similar – type 4)

It was possible to compare two types of rehabilitation programmes and thus a type 4 design was also an option. For the evaluation users – managers, professionals and those paying for the progammes – one question of interest would be whether it is worth setting up work-based rehabilitation programmes as an alternative to the traditional primary care programmes.

6 Can you compare the intervention to comparison or a placebo and randomise (for better control)? (type 5)

In principle it would have been possible to randomise patients to the multidisciplinary programme and to the other programme or a placebo and hence a type 5 design was also an option. But would this design have better answered the users' questions than the type 4 or 3 designs? Do we already know whether the multidisciplinary programme is better than a placebo? Or is our question about the difference in outcome for patients between the multidisciplinary and traditional programmes? There are also practical and financial constraints which make it difficult to get a sufficient number of patients to give statistically significant results.

7 Can you compare before and after for intermediate targets? (type 6a)

The type 6 design is for evaluating interventions to organisations such as a training programme. This design was not appropriate for the rehabilitation example because the evaluation was of the effects of rehabilitation on patients as targets, not, for example, of the effect of a training programme on personnel.

8 Can you compare before and after for final targets? (type 6b)

This also was not an appropriate design for the rehabilitation programme for the reasons given above.

The above questions help to consider the usefulness of each design for answering the users' questions. When planning how to evaluate something, consider which designs you could use and then look at the time and money you have and decide which is feasible. It is not a waste of time to consider the ideal design even if you do not have the time and money to carry it out; awareness of the ideal makes it easier to describe the limitations of the design which you do choose and also gives ideas about how to make up for these limitations when planning your study.

> *If you want certainty, try religion. Evaluation at best will give data to reduce uncertainty and to help make decisions. Spending more money and time on the evaluation can increase the certainty of the findings, but how certain do users need to be to make the decision?*

Different designs would answer different questions and some designs are more expensive and take longer than others. Whether the extra time and cost are worth it depends on for whom we are doing the evaluation and their questions. An RCT may be too expensive and take too long for some users or may not be practical or ethical. Evaluations are to help people make better informed decisions than they would otherwise do.

Once the type of design is decided, the evaluator has to consider the details of design which include:

- which data need to be collected about the intervention, environment, targets and outcomes?
- are these data already available or do they need to be specially collected?
- how accurate do the different data need to be for the users' decisions?

Collecting data takes time and money and analysing the data can take even more: data collection and analysis is the main resource demand in an evaluation. The three factors which have the biggest resource implications for the evaluator are:

- the amount of data required about outcomes (one measure or many measures?) and about the targets and context (if these are changing)
- the length of time over which data are collected and the frequency of collection
- whether a comparison control is required (which doubles the data collection and calls for data to check similarities).

In the rehabilitation example, many data about outcomes and the targets were collected, leaving less time and money to collect data about the intervention and aspects of the environment. Did the evaluators get the balance wrong?

Initial questions for analysing or planning an evaluation

There are some basic questions to ask when reading a report of an evaluation or when starting to design your own evaluation study. These are questions about the purpose of the evaluation. We can take the example of the rehabilitation programme evaluation to illustrate these. The initial questions to ask of this and of most evaluations are as follows.

- Who was or is the evaluation for – the primary evaluation users? (e.g. Is it for the management of an organisation, for health practitioners, for government policy makers or for a patients' association?)
- Which questions does it aim to answer? (e.g. What are the effects of the intervention on health? Is the cost of the intervention worth the benefits?)
- Which decisions and actions should be better informed as a result? What do people need to know to act differently or to do with more confidence what they do now (e.g. a decision about whether to continue the programme or to extend it to others)?

And, for designing your own evaluation:

- How much time and resources are available? (when are the results required, how much of your and others' time is available, which other resources do you need such as computer software or access to statistical expertise?)

Other starting questions include:

- Which perspective should be taken to assess the value of the intervention? (e.g. just the perspective of managers, the perspective of employees or the perspective of the community? The more perspectives which are included, then the more expensive and complicated the evaluation.)
- What are the key value criteria by which the evaluation users will judge the value of the intervention? This refers to what is important to people: in the example, the values appear to be the ability to work and symptom reduction.

Box 10.2: Questions to ask to analyse or design an evaluation

- User? Who is the evaluation for and which user perspective to take?
- Intervention? What is the service, action or change to be evaluated?
- Target? Who or what does the intervention aim to change?
- Which value criteria? How do the users judge the value of the intervention?
- What do users need to know to change what they do now or to make better informed decisions?
- Outcomes of interest? Which data to collect to find out if the targets changed or to discover other changes?
- Confounders? What could explain the outcomes, apart from the intervention?

Summary

- How do you know if an evaluation is good or bad? How do you decide whether to act on the findings? A quick way to assess any evaluation is to use the '4D' method to score the description of the intervention, and the quality of data about outcomes, targets and the intervention environment, the appropriateness of the design and the decision relevance for your work or organisation.
- Evaluation is a service to a user and the best evaluation design is the one which best meets their needs within the constraints of the study.
- The main considerations in deciding which design to use are the informational needs of the evaluation user, the scope of the outcome data required (in time and breadth), the resources and timescale available and the skills available to the evaluators.

- One way to choose which design to use is to work through the following questions about features of the intervention, target and the environment.
  - How controllable are the intervention and confounders?
  - How specific and stable is the intervention and how controllable are other confounders such as target characteristics and context?
  - Can you describe the intervention? (if not, type 1 design is useful)
  - Can you compare the intentions to what was done? Are objectives or procedures specified? (if yes, then type 2 design can be used)
  - Can you compare targets before and after? (if yes, then type 3 is possible)
  - Can you compare to control (nothing or similar)? (if yes, then type 4 is possible)
  - Can you compare to control and randomise (for better control)? (if yes, then type 5 is possible if you have the resources)
  - Can you compare before and after for intermediate targets? (type 6a)
  - Can you compare before and after for final targets? (type 6b)

Specific subjects

Part 3 of the book discusses specific subjects in detail. It considers data-gathering methods, the politics and ethics of evaluation, quality evaluation and evaluation paradigms and perspectives.

Chapter 11

Data-gathering methods

Introduction

Of all the things which evaluators do, data gathering is the most visible and takes up the most time. Yet in some ways it is the least important. Whilst it does require some skill and resourcefulness, data gathering itself is fairly routine. It is planning which data to collect before and data analysis after which take the time and skill. Data analysis often takes longer than it should because the evaluator has not defined clearly which questions the data need to answer and has not done sufficient planning work in the pre-data collection phases of the evaluation described in Chapter 4.

This is one reason why data gathering is not discussed in detail earlier in the text: if the planning work, especially defining who the evaluation users are and their value criteria, is well done, then data gathering and analysis are much quicker and less demanding and fewer data are wasted. Another reason is that many of the methods are familiar to anyone with a research background.

Carrying out an evaluation is likely to require us to use methods which we have not used before or may not even know about. Our 'home disciplines' favour particular data-gathering methods which are suited to the subject of the discipline. We may be unfamiliar with or suspicious about the methods used by other disciplines and which we may need to use in an evaluation. Evaluators need to be broad-minded about methods and knowledgeable about a number of ways to gather data. Users of evaluations need to understand how the data were produced and analysed in order to judge the validity of the conclusions.

Some of the questions considered are as follows.

- Do you have to use measures in an evaluation?
- Should you use qualitative or quantitative methods?
- How can you collect qualitative information in a way that makes it easier to analyse it and is credible to others?
- How do you gather valid data about an intervention or about the people who may be affected by it?

The chapter does not discuss data gathering in detail because there are many other texts which give excellent descriptions of different data-gathering methods and these are noted in the course of the discussion. Rather, it gives a simple introduction to five categories of method: using already collected data (such as government statistics); observation; interviewing; questionnaires and surveying; and specific measurement methods.

After reading this chapter you should be:

- able to describe the five categories of data-gathering methods and know how to obtain more details about how to use them
- more willing to use methods you are not familiar with, if these data can give evidence about the intervention you are interested in
- more questioning about what should be considered as 'evidence'
- better able to recognise the limitations of the methods used in an evaluation, invalid and unreliable data or whether evaluators have not used the methods properly.

Data gathering

Data gathering describes a part of the evaluation where the evaluator identifies sources of data, gets access to these sources and collects necessary data. It describes a range of methods within the following five categories.

- *Already collected data*: data collected for other purposes, by a service, government departments, other researchers, opinion polls and other people (e.g. journalists) ('secondary data'), as well as diary records, minutes of meetings, patient case records, legal documents, etc. (sometimes called 'primary sources').
- *Observation*: unobtrusive, participant or self-observation.
- *Interviews*: structured (e.g. questions), semi-structured, open or guided by a critical incident or vignette stimulus. Focus group interviews.
- *Questionnaire or survey*: small- or large-scale survey, with or without rating scales.
- *Measurement methods*: biophysical, subjective response or a pre-formulated measurement instrument such as disease-specific or quality of life composite measures.

What is 'evidence'?

The terms 'data gathering' or 'collection' imply that facts 'lie around' waiting to be collected by a 'scientific vacuum cleaner'. This is not the view taken by this book, which does not see facts as existing independently of an observer. But neither does it regard facts as being entirely constructed by the mind of the observer; data 'production' or 'creation' would also be slightly misleading ways to describe data gathering.

The view taken here is that facts are created in a relationship between the observer and the observed in interaction and through relationships between observers who agree what is to be counted a fact and how to gather factual information (inter-subjective agreement about procedures). Facts and evidence do not exist without the method for 'gathering' or 'creating' them or without pre-observational categories. Whether data are 'valid evidence' depends on the method being used in the right way, using techniques to maximise validity and reliability which have been developed for that method. Data from measurement techniques such as a blood pressure instrument are not more or less valid than data from interviews.

Before discussing each category of methods, there are a few final introductory points to be made about how the methods are used within an evaluation study.

The way a data-gathering method is used depends on the perspective of the research. An experimentalist approach will use data collection to test hypotheses and will have carefully pre-defined concepts and measures. A subjectivist or phenomenological study (described in Chapter 14) will work more inductively, building up concepts and hypotheses out of the data. Both perspectives may use interviewing or observation, but will be using these data-gathering methods in different ways.

Some methods are termed 'quantitative' because they assign numbers to an aspect of a person, organisation or event. 'Qualitative' data-gathering methods, on the other hand, are ways of recording and understanding people's experiences and the meanings which they give to events and their behaviour in natural settings (Pope and Mays, 1995b). For simplicity, this chapter follows the traditional terminology of describing methods as 'qualitative' or 'quantitative', even though these terms should be applied to data, not to the methods. Some methods, such as interviewing, can be used to gather data in a qualitative or quantitative form.

Qualitative data are often gathered as part of an inductive approach, which seeks to build up categories of meaning out of the data, usually from people's reported experiences and perceptions or observations of their behaviour. In this way the researcher defines categories of meaning after and sometimes during data collection, rather than before. 'Qualitative evaluation' is evaluation which only uses qualitative methods. For some purposes this gives more valid data than quantitative methods, but these data may be less reliable.

We can only assess the suitability of a data-gathering method in relation to the particular questions and informational needs of the user. Thus there is no such thing as the 'general validity' of a measure or data-gathering method, only validity in relation to a particular purpose.

Box 11.1: Eight golden rules of data collection

1 Don't collect data unless you are sure no one else has already done so.
2 Don't invent a new measure when a proven one will do.
3 When the person or documents you need to see are not available, don't ignore what is available which could help – be opportunistic.
4 Measure what's important, not what's easy to measure.
5 Don't collect data where confounders make interpretation impossible.
6 Spend twice as much time on planning and designing the evaluation as you spend on data collection.
7 Analysing the data takes twice as long as collecting them, if you have not defined clearly which data you need and why.
8 Data collection will take twice long as you expect.

Using existing data sources

'Existing data' are data already collected for purposes other than the evaluation and include government statistics, hospital or primary care centre administrative data and patient records. Here we will consider both the methods which are commonly used to collect these data and the methods which evaluators can use to find, abstract and analyse them.

Before using already collected data, be careful to check how they were collected and whether you can use them for the evaluation. The main problems are finding out if any data already exist which you might be able to use and then discovering how the data were collected and recorded. We need to know which methods were used in order to judge the validity and reliability of the data and to decide if we can use the data for our purposes.

Identify data sources

The first step is to identify possible sources of already collected data, called 'secondary sources'. As with all data collection methods, this depends on being clear about which types of evidence are required to answer the evaluation question and which would give evidence in relation to the evaluation criteria. Is evidence needed about the outcomes of the service, policy or organisational change or about processes or inputs? And what type of evidence: patient perceptions, staff perceptions, economic or other types of evidence? Over what timescale is the evidence required? Answers to these questions help to suggest possible sources of existing data.

There are different ways of searching for sources. The simplest is to ask service providers or clerical staff if there are records, statistics and other sources which might give the data needed for the evaluation. Sometimes it is easier to ask patients what they think that service providers might have recorded or whether any patients have kept a diary. The evaluator can also look at public or private indexes or registers of documents held by institutions. For identifying data already published in research reports and journals there are a variety of databases and search methods such as MEDLINE and Social Science Citations Indexes.

Service statistics include data about inputs and processes such as bed numbers, admissions, staffing and sometimes data about outcomes. Health service activity and performance data include: numbers referred, numbers using the service, numbers discharged, age and sex and other patient characteristics, types of needs/diagnoses, types and numbers of treatments provided, throughput, bed utilisation, average length of treatment, waiting lists, waiting times, unit costs, staffing numbers/ grades, absenteeism, sickness and turnover. Some countries also have national or local statistics on number of patients for the major diagnostic-related groups (DRGs).

There are also individual case records and these are already used for some types of evaluation such as some quality assurance procedures or audit. Medical and other types of audit reports are also useful data sources for some evaluations (e.g. NCEPOD, 1987, 1989, 1993).

Assessing the data

The second step in this method is to assess the data for the purposes of the evaluation. This means applying the same tests to these already recorded data which one applies to data gathered using a direct method such as an interview or questionnaire. The tests include validity, reliability, sampling and tests of appropriate analysis if the data are already presented as composite measures. If comparing two services or sites, it is necessary to check that the available data were collected in the same way. Note, however, that these tests should be applied to the data relative to the degree of certainty which evaluation users require for their decisions.

A separate issue to consider in assessing the potential use of the data source is the question of confidentiality. There are usually strict rules to ensure patient confidentiality which evaluators will need to understand and respect. Some evaluators have found that these rules become even stricter when service providers hear that the records are needed for an evaluation.

Using the data

The third step is to abstract from the data sources those data necessary for the evaluation and to analyse them. The data may be qualitative, as for example in descriptions in case records or in minutes or agendas of meetings. If so, the evaluator uses coding or other methods of abstraction and data analysis for qualitative data, always bearing in mind that the text was recorded for purposes other than the evaluation. Often the evaluator uses already collected quantitative data and analyses them using statistical and other methods, depending on their assessment as described above.

In my experience the detective work in discovering already collected data is well worth the effort, especially if these data pass the assessment described above. Sometimes discovering that there are no recorded data is itself an important finding. For example, in an evaluation of total quality programmes in six Norwegian hospitals, one finding was that there was little documentation of the quality projects which were running and few of these projects were using measures, despite documentation, reporting and measurement being generally agreed as essential features of such programmes (Øvretveit, 1999). Discovering that there are recorded data but that they are not available to the evaluator or cannot be made public is itself useful information for an evaluation.

Observation

Observation methods are used to collect data about the behaviour of people. The people may be patients or people providing a service or implementing a policy or other people such as carers, voluntary workers or politicians. 'Behaviour' is what people do and say.

Observation can be carried out by using a pre-structured coded observation form or by 'open' observation and both these methods may be used by an independent observer or by a participant observer. One particularly useful method for gaining data about a service process is to observe and record what happens to a patient as the researcher follows them in their 'journey' from admission to discharge or beyond (a 'Tracer patient pathway study'; Øvretveit, 1994b). This can be combined with interviewing the patient to gather their perceptions at different stages.

If used within a qualitative paradigm, 'open' observation allows evaluators skilled in this method to study what people do in a natural setting and to build up a conceptualisation which reflects people's behaviour in this setting. The aim here is not to impose pre-defined categories and 'count' behaviour, as would be the approach using this method within an experimental paradigm, but to 'suspend' the observer's categories and to carefully record what is observed in 'field notes'. The aim is to observe and record as faithfully and factually as possible, for example by recording the words used rather than summaries. This can necessitate video or audio recording, although this can influence people's actions even more than the presence of the observer.

Participant observation is a method which reduces the influence of the observer on people's behaviour but requires the participant observer to take part in everyday life for some time, sometimes without disclosing their role as an observer. This increases validity but still leaves a question as to whether a similarly trained observer would see and record the same things. There are also ethical problems with the participant observer role; for example, some view it as deliberate deception and betraying the trust of patients and healthcare workers.

Strengths and weaknesses

The strengths of observation methods are that they give direct evidence of observed outcomes and processes, rather than reported accounts. Data from observation can be used to develop theories about how the context affects behaviour and why people react as they do. Observation also gives real examples for a research report which capture the flavour of the setting. But whilst there are some uses for this method, there are four 'threats' to validity which make it a less attractive method for those who are not trained anthropologists or sociologists. First, there are problems in ensuring the reliability of observations so that valid comparisons can be made. Second, the effect of the observer on what people do is likely to be greater if the people know that the observer is an evaluator: every child knows that teacher acts differently when the school inspector is there. Third, pre-coded observation categories, if they are used, may ignore the different meanings of the same behaviour in different places.

The fourth threat to validity applies to the use of this method within a qualitative paradigm where the observer does not use pre-set categories. How do we know whether the observer imposes their own categories or 'distorts' what they observe? The observer has to have some categories or ways of seeing to decide what to observe and record – there is no such thing as 'unbiased observation'. Qualitative researchers recognise these criticisms and have a number of strategies to reduce observer bias and increase validity. They emphasise that the categories are built up inductively and stress the ideal of factual description; that records provide evidence which can be checked by others, including the participants ('participant validation'); and that multiple observers are used and that observation is one of multiple sources of data ('triangulation'; Jick, 1983).

These and other problems and details of the observational method in conventional health research are described in outline in McConway (1994, pp. 22–6, with examples from bedside medical teaching), Pope and Mays (1995a, b, pp. 182–4) and in more detail in Sapsford and Abbott (1992, pp. 127–35). Practical general accounts are given in Edwards and Talbot (1994, pp. 76–85), and how to use pre-coded observation is described in Breakwell and Millward (1995). More detailed discussions can be found in general texts on social science methods, such as Adams and Shvaneveldt (1991).

Interviewing

Interviewing gives the evaluator access to people's views, their recollected experiences, feelings and their theories about causation. This method can be used to collect data in a quantitative form, where the interviewer uses pre-structured categories and questions (e.g. a pre-coded questionnaire administered in an interview). It can also be used to collect qualitative data by using open-ended questions or a set of topics for open exploration and probing by the interviewer. Here we consider interviewing as a method for collecting qualitative data, used within a qualitative paradigm.

In-depth interviewing can be semi-structured, with a set of topics, or unstructured where the interviewer is led by the person's concerns and aims to discover what a person's views are and why they hold these views. Interviewing of this type is a skilled task requiring the interviewer to demonstrate interest without becoming overinvolved and biased, to gain trust, to appear neutral and non-judgemental and to know when and how to probe when something of general interest to the research arises. There is a 'therapeutic' dimension to interviewing in evaluations, which is considered later. During some research, interviewers may change their interview strategies so as to pursue topics and hypotheses which have emerged out of previous interviews.

Interviews are useful for gaining data about patients' experiences, in their own terms. Interviews can elicit patients' recollected experiences, for example of their situation and expectations before undergoing a treatment. Interviews also allow the evaluator to discover how health service personnel understood or responded to an intervention or a policy. These are important data for understanding how or why some policies work or fail; the perceptions of staff and their reasons for acting in the way they do can be useful data for all types of evaluation. A policy or change often has a meaning or symbolic importance which is not recognised by outsiders, but may be critical to the impact of an intervention; this is as true for interventions into health services as it is for health education programmes for particular groups. How people interpret change is important for understanding its effects and interviews are the main way of gathering data about how people interpret and understand interventions. The evaluator can build theories about how an intervention works or fails, either by testing their own theories in interviews or by seeking out and refining participants' theories.

Before considering the strengths and weaknesses of interview methods for comparative research, we will consider one type of group interview.

Focus group interview method

The advantage of an 'interview' with a group rather than with individuals is the ability to gain a range of views more quickly and with fewer resources than a series of interviews. The focus group technique is one form of group interview where the 'facilitator-interviewer' leads a group of about eight people in a discussion of a particular topic. As with individual interviews, there may be an agenda or the facilitator may allow the discussion to develop with little prompting or probing or may give example situations (e.g. 'critical incidents') or vignettes to stimulate views. If the group members have similar backgrounds then they usually feel less inhibited but this may mean that the research will need many different focus groups to ensure that a range of views is captured.

When people are in a group with 'similar' people they are usually less intimidated by the interviewer and may speak more openly and stimulate each other to recall different incidents and express views. However, it is often less easy in a group to probe and follow up one person's views and also there may be a greater pressure to express views which a person thinks are acceptable to the group (group conformity). For example, Kitzinger (1995) notes:

> *In group discussion with old people in residential care I found that some residents tried to prevent others from criticising staff – becoming agitated and repeatedly interrupting with cries of 'You can't complain', 'The staff couldn't possibly be nicer'.*

The quality of the data depends even more than with individual interviews on the skills of the facilitator, and detailed recording is more difficult, although video or tape recording may be possible.

Summaries of focus group technique in health services can be found in Fitzpatrick and Boulton (1994, p. 108) and Kitzinger (1995, pp. 299–302). More details are given by Morgan (1993, e.g. when to use focus groups and why, pp. 3–19) and by Kreuger (1988). An example of focus group technique in peer service quality research is given in Øvretveit (1991a) and its use in patient satisfaction research in Øvretveit (1992b).

Strengths and weaknesses of interview methods

Qualitative interviewing is a method for discovering peoples' experiences, the meaning of events to them, their feelings or their 'lay theories'. But, as with observation, there are drawbacks and problems of validity and reliability for evaluation. Would a similarly trained interviewer have gathered the same data? How does one analyse pages of interview transcript and how would an evaluation user judge whether the conclusions were really based on the interview data or whether the interviewer biased the subjects' responses? How can we ensure consistency between interviewers?

To some extent interviews create data in the sense that interviewees often have not thought about the issues on which they are questioned. Interviewees usually do not simply report their experiences, but they create or make more explicit what they think during the interview. The skill of the interviewer is to enable the person to reflect on and develop their ideas, without introducing the interviewer's own biases. A second validity issue is that the interviewee may not recollect 'properly' or may have a selective view of the event. Golden (1992) describes work which shows that managers recollect with 'hindsight bias' and in ways which unconsciously maintain their own self-esteem; she describes methods to reduce this bias and emphasises the need to acknowledge the limitations of such data.

A third validity issue is that interviewees may be more concerned with projecting the right image and how they appear rather than with representing 'the truth'. For example, men reported about 30% higher levels of morbidity when they were interviewed by women than they did when interviewed by men (Nathanson, 1978). As with observation, triangulation and corroboration can be used to increase validity, as well as probing where people give discrepant accounts, and 'respondent validation' can be used to check emerging analyses with the people interviewed or with another group.

Investigating sensitive or 'difficult' topics with interviewing raises ethical issues. Techniques to put the interviewee at ease, to encourage them to 'open up' and empathising methods are recommended in some texts and taught in training programmes for interviewers and qualitative researchers. There can be problems when these techniques are used with patients or health service staff who have had a bad or traumatic experience, for example to investigate poor quality or disasters.

In these situations the researcher may be the only person to whom the patient or staff member has talked about the experience and the researcher is using powerful techniques which will encourage the interviewee to reawaken their experience. The researcher then goes off with their data, leaving the interviewee to cope with what has been evoked in the interview. I have known some well-meaning qualitative studies where junior researchers have not been able to deal with the feelings of distress uncovered by these techniques. Talking about an experience does not of itself cure the original trauma; more is required to help a person work through an experience after being 'opened up'. Planners need to recognise the 'therapeutic' dimension of interviewing, the ethical issues and the need for appropriate interviewer supervision.

A strength of some interview methods is that they allow the researcher to build up an understanding of the patients' and healthcare providers' experiences, meanings and feelings, by understanding people in their own settings and on their own terms. This is particularly important for gathering data about outcomes and about how interventions may work where people's feelings are an important mediating variable. Problems of validity are similar to those above: the researcher may impose their own biases and categories rather than represent those of the participants; interviews often create as much as they reflect people's views; problems arise in reporting the analysis and conclusions;

there are difficulties in knowing how general the findings might be; and problems arise in reliability or replication.

Both observation and interviewing can be used to collect data in a quantitative or qualitative form. When choosing a data-gathering method, the researcher needs to consider how they will analyse the data and present it to users. One of the greatest weaknesses of qualitative observation and interviewing is the difficulty in analysing and presenting the data, especially to users who are unfamiliar with or sceptical of these methods.

For more details of qualitative open interviewing in health settings the reader is referred to a summary in Britten (1995, pp. 251–3), Sapsford and Abbott (1992, pp. 108–15), McConway (1994, pp. 27–30, who also introduces 'feminism and qualitative interviewing' in healthcare) and Fitzpatrick and Boulton (1994, pp. 107–8). Practical summaries are given by Edwards and Talbot (1994, pp. 86–9) and Breakwell and Millward (1995, pp. 67–73). One interesting example of the use of semi-structured interviewing is given in a study which sought older people's perceptions of care and problems (Powell *et al.*, 1994). The in-depth interview method in organisational studies is described in Ghauri *et al.* (1995, pp. 64–72). General social science methodology texts give extensive practical and theoretical discussion of the method. Kvale (1994) gives a very readable and concise discussion of 'ten standard objections to qualitative research interviews'.

Surveying and questionnaires

Asking questions is one way of finding out what people think about a particular topic and we saw above how this could be done using a semi-structured interview method. Another method is a self-completed questionnaire, which can be mailed or completed by a person when they are in hospital, receiving care or at work. Examples of these methods include large-scale population surveys with pre-set categories and questionnaires designed to discover patients' expectations and experiences of treatment.

Questionnaires are used when evaluators want to collect data about specific topics and where the topics have the same meaning and are well understood by people in different settings or social groups. Questionnaires are less expensive than interviews, which are unnecessary where simple factual data are required or where people can easily and authentically express their ideas in terms of the categories used by the researcher in the questionnaire. Questionnaires can gather qualitative data by asking people to write descriptive accounts. More often, questionnaires use one or more measurement scales which thus provide quantitative data.

The best-known scales are the Likert five-item scale and a semantic differential scale (pairs of opposites, e.g. painful–not painful, usually with a seven-point scale) (see Breakwell and Millward, 1995, pp. 64–6 for a simple summary). Again this can be a source of biased data, for example where people from different cultures use the extremes of rating scales in a different way (Van De Vijver and Leung, 1997). The way the questions are worded and their order are important to validity. Of particular importance in design is to look ahead to how the analysis will be performed and with quantitative questionnaires (e.g. with rating scales) issues such as sample size need to be considered if statistically valid inferences are to be drawn from the data.

Strengths and weaknesses

The advantages of questionnaires are that they allow people time to think and to respond anonymously. They are quick and easy to analyse (if there are few 'open questions' and they are pre-coded) and they can be given to many people at a low cost. A disadvantage is that it can be difficult to get a high response rate (over 50%) and questionnaires may be returned by a disproportionate number of people who feel particularly strongly about a topic (selective response rate), which can give misleading results if the researcher generalises the findings without noting this possibility. Other disadvantages include a proportion only being partly-completed and some respondents may 'misuse' or misunderstand the categories or feel that they cannot express their view properly in the terms required. People from different ethnic groups use the extremes of scales differently (Van De Vijver and Leung, 1997). Some subjects may under- or overestimate in their replies. For example, McKinlay (1992) found that questionnaire respondents generally under-reported their alcohol consumption by about half, although he also notes that this under-reporting is even greater when respondents are interviewed.

The most well-known problem is the different responses with different question phrasing or use of terms, which adds a further complication to crosscultural studies. For example, US opinion polls found that 55% of people said that they would vote for a law allowing the terminally ill to choose 'euthanasia'. This rate increased to 65% when the question was rephrased to ask whether they would support the right of the terminally ill to choose 'death with dignity' over prolonging life. Forty four percent would allow a terminally ill person to choose a 'lethal injection' but 50%

would approve a 'medical procedure'. Another UK study asking questions about primary care accidentally found that over half the respondents thought primary care meant care which was more important or urgent and about 35% thought that secondary care was lower quality care. Much depends on the skill and experience of the questionnaire designer!

These and other issues are discussed in detail in general texts (e.g. Frankfort-Nachmias and Nachmias, 1992) and research texts (e.g. Breakwell and Millward, 1995, pp. 58–67). Questionnaire design is summarised in McConway (1994, pp. 57–8), Sapsford and Abbott (1992, pp. 87–100) and Edwards and Talbot (1994, pp. 99–101). McKinlay (1992, pp. 115–37) gives an excellent discussion of methods used for surveying older people. Surveys and questionnaires for organisational research are discussed in Ghauri *et al.* (1995, pp. 58–64). Hawe *et al.* (1990) describe surveying for evaluating health promotion programmes.

There is a fine dividing line between a questionnaire survey and standard measurement instruments such as the General Health Questionnaire (Bowling, 1992). The difference is that the latter are usually constructed on the basis of an explicit conceptual model and have been extensively tested and often validated, whereas questionnaires and surveys are usually developed for the specific purpose of the research and might have little pilot testing or no validation.

Measurement methods

> *The design of controlled experimentation has been refined to a science that is within the grasp of any researcher who owns a table of random digits and recognises the difference between blind and sighted assessments. However, the measurement of outcome seems to have been abandoned at a primitive stage of development . . . A superfluity of instruments exists, and too little is known about them to prefer one to another. (Smith et al., 1980)*

The above critical view of outcome measures is an extreme one and measures have advanced considerably since 1980. However, it is still true that some evaluators do not choose the most appropriate measure for the purpose of the evaluation and resources available.

Measurement methods are the fifth category of data collection methods considered here. When used as a general term, 'measurement' describes any method of data collection; questionnaires are sometimes described as measures. Here the term is used in a specific sense to mean only methods for collecting data in a numerical or 'quantified' form. More precisely, measurement is assigning numerical values to objects, events or empirical facts according to specified rules. In this sense we may measure a person's attitude by asking them to express their views in terms of a number on a rating scale (an ordinal scale) or measure their temperature using a thermometer (a ratio scale). We gather data not about the entity or the concept but about the properties of a concept. This involves using indicators which are observable events that are inferred measures of concepts.

Measurement quantifies something by comparison with something else. Measures are often used in research to quantify needs and outcome, but also to quantify inputs (e.g. costing) and processes (e.g. time, the number of defined activities). Measurement is an efficient way to communicate evidence and describe things.

In evaluations there are three types of phenomena which are often quantified:

- physical states, such as death and disease, or events such as the number of hospital beds or nurses
- activities, practices and processes, such as length of stay, financing methods and quality systems
- perceptions and attitudes, such as employees' views about a new policy and attitudes towards a new treatment.

Measures of patient outcomes used in treatment and service research include measures of physiological functioning (temperature, blood pressure, haemoglobin value, erythrocyte sedimentation rate, glucose levels, etc.), measures of physical function (e.g. activities of daily living, ability to walk, range of motion), measures of psychological functioning (e.g. response rate, cognitive abilities, depression, anxiety) and measures of social functioning (e.g. social skills, ability to participate in employment, community participation, etc.).

For some evaluations we use numbers and a denominator, such as 'X per 100 000 population', which are termed 'rates' (the ratio of two measures). Some comparisons are in terms of composite measures, such as a composite measure for mortality which includes infant and maternal mortality and possibly other mortality rates. Such measures are sometimes called indices or indicators, where a number of different indicators are brought together in a formula to produce one number which is then compared.

This section does not describe these different measures in detail because they are well described in general research texts such as Bowling's texts on measuring disease (Bowling, 1995) and her review of quality of life measures (Bowling, 1992) as well as in research texts such as Fink (1993), Rossi and Freeman (1993), St Leger *et al.* (1992) and Breakwell and Millward (1995).

> *We value what we measure, so we must learn to measure what we value.*

Concepts and theories underlying measures

When we measure, we or our subjects assign a number to a category – for example, age or a rating of 4 on a scale of 1–5. Or we read off a number from a measuring instrument such as a clock, thermometer or EEG machine. The numbers do not exist before our measurement but are created by us, our subjects or our machines according to certain procedures. These procedures depend on a concept about the phenomenon to which a person using the procedure assigns numbers. The concept of age is one which is commonly agreed and can be measured directly; it is easy to 'operationalise' the concept in the measure of time since birth and everyone knows what it means. Note that this measure itself depends on other concepts and the measure of time. Note also that when we considered qualitative data gathering above we faced issues of operationalisation, for example difficulties in defining a term so that people understood the same thing (e.g. 'illness' or 'quality programme').

Many evaluation criteria are difficult to operationalise (for example, 'health') and we use indicators or proxy measures where the link between the concept and the measure is less direct than for concepts such as age.

Much health research uses numerical data from measures to describe or to explain. Numbers are efficient ways of describing phenomena and allow us to see patterns when they are presented in a visual or graphical way, for example in a pie chart, histogram or scattergram. We can also describe by showing features of the numbers (which hopefully 'represent' features of the phenomenon measured) such as average and spread (e.g. standard deviation, variance, interquartile range). We can see quickly, for example, how many people who received the treatment were within different age ranges or what proportion of the costs of a service was spent on personnel. Numbers also can allow us to discover and prove causation; we consider statistical analysis below.

Generally, most numerical data gathering assumes that:

- the quality or property is sufficiently important to be measured
- the method of measurement can distinguish in a useful way different amounts of the property

- the property of one item at one time can be compared to the property at another time or of another item
- the difference between, for example, 2 and 3 is equal in amount to the difference between 13 and 14 if we are using an interval or ratio scale.

Box 11.2: Some common measurement terms

Sample: a smaller number of a larger population

Prevalence: at a particular time, the number of existing cases identified or arising in a population

Incidence: over a period of time, the number of new cases or events identified or arising in a population

Rate: a ratio of two measures, such as the proportion of a population with a particular problem or characteristic, often expressed by age or by sex (e.g. cases out of 100 000). Rates require data from interval or ratio scales.

Prevalence rate is the proportion of cases in a population at a particular time (e.g. 26 in 100 000).

Incidence rate is the proportion of new cases which arise over a period of time. Death or mortality rate is the proportion of a population who die during a defined time period

---

Analysing data

Having gathered data about the intervention and probably the outcomes and targets, the evaluator then will need to analyse these data. In this section we briefly note methods for analysing data in quantitative and qualitative forms.

Quantitative data analysis

Any data produced using measures will have errors. Some of the errors will be produced by the measurement method and may be chance errors or systematic bias. Increasing the sample size will not reduce systematic bias in the measuring method. However, some variation is inherent in the item being studied and is not an artifact of the method. Statistical techniques are used to minimise variation and to analyse data which includes variation. Techniques for calculating statistical significance and confidence intervals help researchers and users to assess the probability of associations and to make inferences about causes.

Box 11.3: Terms used in quantitative data analysis

Internal validity: the validity of the conclusions in relation to the specific sample of the study. For example, in an evaluation experiment, being able to show whether or not the intervention has an effect or the size of the effect

External validity: the ability of a study to show that the findings would also apply to similar populations, organisations or situations. For example, when an intervention is applied in another setting

Dependent variable: the outcome variable or end result of a treatment, service or policy which is the subject of the study (e.g. cancer mortality, patient satisfaction, resources consumed by a service) and which might be associated with or even caused by other (independent) variables. (The data analysis tests for associations between the dependent (outcome) variable and the independent variables. Establishing causation is more complex.)

Independent variable(s): a variable whose possible effect on the dependent variable is examined. Something which may cause the outcome and which is tested in the research. (Note: Many independent variables may be associated with a dependent variable, but only a few have a causal influence and even fewer can be shown unambiguously to have a causal effect. A dependent variable cannot influence an independent variable, e.g. genetic make-up can predispose to cancer but cancer, as far as we know, cannot affect genes.)

Mediating variable(s): other variables which could affect the dependent variable or outcome, which the research tries to control for in design or in statistical analysis

Extraneous variable(s): variables not considered in the theory or model used in the study

Confounding variable(s): any variable which influences the dependent variable or outcome but was not considered or controlled for in the study. Alternative definition: 'confounding arises when an observed association between two variables is due to the action of a third factor' (Crombie, 1996)

In many evaluations we have two sets of numbers, for example a 'before' and an 'after' set, or outcomes from two services in different places. Statistical significance testing helps to show whether or not any differences between the two sets really represent true differences in the populations from which the samples were drawn. It is based on the idea that any difference between the two sets is caused by a real difference as well as by differences arising from random and systematic error introduced by the measurement method. It involves proposing a null hypothesis – that there is no difference between the sets – and examining whether any difference shown is greater than that expected by chance. The significance level is the level of probability at which we decide to reject the null hypothesis.

> *What is meant by statistically significant? It simply means that it did not occur by chance alone, there is probably some external cause . . . It does not prove that the variables being investigated caused the difference . . . It is up to the researcher to prove that the variables under consideration are the actual cause and to eliminate the possibility of any other variable(s) contributing to the results found.* (Black, 1992)

Phillips *et al.* (1994) give a useful and simple summary of the main statistical methods for analysis by distinguishing different stages of analysis. The first is to describe and summarise the data by representing each numerical value in a pie chart or bar chart, by calculating the averages (the mean, median and mode), the range (the difference between the smallest and largest value in a data set) and the standard deviation (how much the data values deviate from the average). The second stage is to define the generalisability of the data by stating how much confidence we would have of finding the results from the sample in the general population. This is done by calculating the 'confidence interval'. A third hypothesis-testing stage involves using data to confirm or reject a hypothesis. A type 1 error is rejection of a null hypothesis when it is in fact true: the analysis calculates the probability of having a type 1 error, called the 'significance level'. A fourth stage is to calculate the strength of the association between two variables using chi-squared tests, calculating a correlation coefficient or carrying out a regression analysis.

Giving a short listing of these statistical methods makes them look more complicated than they are. There are now a number of texts which give simple summaries with examples. Techniques for deciding significance levels and other details of measurement, sampling and statistical analysis in health research are described in summary in St Leger *et al.* (1992, Chapter 11), Edwards and Talbot (1994, Chapter 6) and

McConway (1994, Chapters 5 and 6). A simple general practical overview of 'describing and summarising data' and of drawing inferences in evaluation is given in Breakwell and Millward (1995, pp. 80–96). Wiltkin *et al.* (1992) describe measurement of need and outcome, as does Bowling (1992, 1995). A more detailed and comprehensive text for clinicians is Gardner and Altman (1989).

Qualitative data analysis

The greatest challenge to using qualitative data in evaluation is analysing the data. The challenge does not stop there: there is the related problem of how to display qualitative data and to convince users and scientists that the conclusions are justified by the data. There are two issues. First, how to use the techniques of analysis which are generally agreed by qualitative researchers in order to reach conclusions which other scientists using these methods would accept. Second, how to present the conclusions and analysis to those who are not familiar with these techniques.

Many people in the health services are familiar with methods for analysing and presenting quantitative data, but not with those for qualitative data. Data analysis is one of the most difficult, time-consuming but also creative tasks in using observation and interviewing methods within a qualitative paradigm. Analysis can be made after the data collection phase, but also during data collection. We noted this technique when describing interview methods, where an interviewer follows up a subject of interest or formulates a hypothesis and explores it through probing and testing within the interview. A similar process of analysis is where the interviewer carries out an analysis after an interview and uses the 'results' in subsequent interviews, these results being categories of experience or hypotheses which can be tested.

We can represent a common approach to qualitative data analysis by the following steps.

- Interview or observation
- Text (a write-up of the interview or field notes or transcript of a tape)
- Code or classify (according to 'emergent' themes or patterns)
- Further analysis (re-coding or hypothesis testing, often by returning to original text or other texts to compare views or settings for similarities and differences)
- Conclusions/results: categories of experience or feelings of the subjects, meanings subjects give to events, explanatory models and concepts or generalisations

Qualitative analysis is inductive, building and testing concepts in interaction with the data or the subjects. It is also usually iterative: the analyst forms categories from the data and then returns to the data to test their generalisability.

These techniques of data analysis are complex and are not easy to describe in research reports for readers unfamiliar with the techniques, but then this is also true for methods for analysing quantitative data. However, examples from the original data give vivid illustrations and also 'ring true' with users. A comprehensive and detailed account of qualitative data analysis is given in Miles and Huberman (1994), but simpler and shorter summaries are provided in Fitzpatrick and Boulton (1994, pp. 110–1), Edwards and Talbot (1994, pp. 102–5) and Sapsford and Abbot (1992, pp. 117–25). A discussion specifically for evaluation is given in Patton (1987). Other good general texts on qualitative data collection methods and philosophy include Denzin and Lincoln (1994), Glaser and Strauss (1968), Greene (1994), Lincoln and Guba (1985), Miles and Huberman (1994), and for reliability and validity tests, Strauss and Corbin (1990).

Summary

- Because of the broad range of subjects and user questions they are faced with, health evaluators need to be aware of a wide range of data-gathering methods.
- Users of evaluations also need to have some understanding of the methods used to gather data in order to judge the validity of the conclusions.
- Data for an evaluation can be collected by methods within the five categories of already collected data, observation, interviewing, questionnaires and surveys, and measurement methods.
- The choice of data-gathering method should follow from the evaluation design and questions to be answered, rather than using the data-gathering method with which the evaluator is most familiar.
- Consider existing data sources: which information is already collected, how accessible is it, and how valid, reliable and comparable is the information for the purposes of the research?
- Never develop a new data-collecting instrument without checking whether you could use an existing and validated instrument (the world does not need another quality of life measure).
- When choosing a method, look ahead to how the data will be analysed and presented. Methods for analysing quantitative data are better

understood in the health sector than methods for analysing qualitative data.

- It is often more difficult to judge the validity of conclusions from qualitative research using participant observation or interview methods than from research using a validated rating scale or measurement instrument.
- Evaluators need to describe the details of the data-gathering methods and the limitations of the data. These details and scrupulous honesty and self-criticism are necessary for others to decide how to use the evaluation and also for the evaluator to develop their skills.
- Some important points to remember are:
  - collecting data costs money
  - a common mistake made by evaluators is to collect more data than they have time to analyse, often because they have not planned beforehand which data they really need
  - collect data which is relevant to the decision
  - does more data make you more certain? Does more accurate data make you more certain? Is the added cost worth the extra certainty?
  - poor data is worse than useless, as it may mislead users to make the wrong decisions.

Chapter 12

The politics and ethics of evaluation

The politics of evaluation are who gains and loses from the evaluation, and how people use an evaluation to advance their interests.

An ethical approach is to be aware of your choices and the consequences and to use ethical principles to choose which course of action to take. The questions are, which ethical principle is the most important in this situation and what could I do to uphold this principle?

The evaluator must be careful not to over-reach the limits of the evaluation and influence decisions which should be made by users or which should be political decisions. There is a fine line in evaluation between being ethical and being political.

Introduction

There is a rude shock awaiting researchers who first undertake an evaluation, thinking it will be like doing research. The shock is to find that they are not welcomed as dispassionate objective scientists by all parties. They are often thrown into a web of intrigue and manoeuvring. Maintaining objectivity is essential, but blind naiveté is not an option for an evaluator. They need to get access to information which may reflect negatively on some people, and many will fear what they will find. Being conscious of the politics of evaluation is important both to the technical outcome of an evaluation but also to acting ethically.

I have carried out more than one evaluation where the organisational culture was not one of openness. People wanted to talk about the programme and found an external evaluator was the only person to whom they could speak openly. On reflection, I became aware that people were reporting serious negligence. Why did they not use the usual channels? If I reported it now it would damage the evaluation, but could patients be harmed if no one took action? Should I just comment about the lack of an effective system for dealing with poor practice and what evidence should I cite to justify my statement?

Evaluator ethics are principles which guide the evaluator in the many difficult situations in which they will find themselves. This chapter continues the theme of Chapter 5 which looked at practical challenges by discussing in more detail the politics of evaluation and by showing how ethics can help both prevent and resolve some of these challenges.

After reading this chapter you should be better able to:

- understand how different parties might respond to your presence as an evaluator and the findings of an evaluation
- prevent common problems by writing a proposal or contract and paying attention to confidentiality, communications and access to the final report
- make use of ethical principles in the heat of the moment as well as to reflect on the best course of action in difficult situations.

The politics of evaluation

The politics of an evaluation are who gains and loses from it, as perceived by different parties. The emphasis here is on their perceptions and feelings; on the need for evaluators to understand how different stakeholders perceive the evaluation process and how they will interpret the findings.

Why are politics an inherent part of evaluation? The link between evaluation and action is closer than for other types of research. If there is no such link, then the evaluation has failed, at least in relation to one criterion of a successful evaluation. The practical consequence of evaluations is often change: practitioners change their practice or finance is reallocated or a policy is extended or cancelled. If there is a change then there are usually winners and losers and a group of people who oppose a change and a group that want it to happen.

Common emotions for people who feel they are being evaluated include fear that their shortcomings will be revealed or that they will be criticised in a way which will damage their interests or self-esteem. Every evaluation has winners and losers, at least in the eyes of the different stakeholders. An understanding of these perceptions and of how different groups will use the evaluation is essential for the evaluator.

The evaluator needs to understand 'unacknowledged agendas' and how to build credibility and trust, how to gain access and co-operation and how best to communicate sensitive findings which could easily be misinterpreted. Both to carry out an evaluation and to maximise the chances of the findings being used, evaluators need to recognise how different groups could be affected by an evaluation. This means understanding how different groups perceive the evaluation both in terms of how it affects them whilst the evaluation is being conducted and how the findings might affect them. Even evaluators who take a detached scientific approach, and who do not accept that they have any responsibility for action, still have to recognise the interests of different groups because these groups can help or hinder their work.

It is important for evaluators and users to think ahead to the possible practical implications of different findings. They need to understand who will gain, lose, be hurt or harmed by the findings. It is best to do this scenario analysis at the planning stage so as to build into the evaluation both practical and technical strategies which will help at later stages. Attention to how an evaluation affects different people is not just for technical purposes – the evaluator has an ethical obligation to consider the impact of what they do and an ethical approach also helps evaluators to negotiate their perilous path.

How, then, do the interests and concerns of different parties affect how the evaluator carries out an evaluation? How does the evaluator anticipate and deal with the politics of evaluation in an ethical way and maintain their integrity? In the following we consider some of the practical issues and possible responses.

> *An evaluation is never scientific enough for the losers. If there are no losers, then the evaluation probably has few practical consequences and is of little value.*

Unacknowledged agendas

There are often reasons why sponsors and others want an evaluation, other than their stated reason. Evaluators need to be aware of 'hidden agendas' before undertaking an evaluation. This helps to think ahead about how to carry out the evaluation and about how their findings will be used, misinterpreted or misused. Managers or others may commission an evaluation as a 'delaying tactic' or to give the impression that something is being done whilst they consider the political options.

The world does not stop for an evaluation: managers have both a right and a duty to consider options, and sometimes to start negotiations, before the results of an evaluation are available. This activity may affect the evaluation; for example, some people may not be willing to provide information if they feel that decisions are already being made. This does not mean that the evaluation is not of use when it is done, but that action may have been 'framed' or even decided before the results are ready.

Other, sometimes unacknowledged reasons for an evaluation are to meet a financing requirement or to increase the chances of a proposal for a new service or intervention being successful. It is becoming more common that services or projects are financed on the condition that the service is evaluated, either externally or has built-in evaluation systems. Proposals are often more likely to be accepted by a financing body if they include a plan to evaluate the proposed project. In these instances the evaluation may be an irrelevant but irritating necessity for those who are successful in their bid to the financing body.

Alternatively, an evaluation may be requested because a politician or a manager has promised that a policy or service will achieve certain objectives and others wish to check whether these promises were met. The evaluator may not know about such promises or commitments and only discover them during the evaluation. They may discover that the aim of one party is to prove the policy or service to be a failure or that promises were not met.

There are limits to how knowledgeable an evaluator can or should be about the motives and intrigues behind a proposed evaluation. In a few circumstances the evaluator should resolutely ignore and stand apart from these issues, as even being aware of them may bias their data gathering or findings. However, in most cases the evaluator needs to ask questions in a diplomatic way about motives and about who wants and does not want the evaluation. They need to be 'streetwise'.

There is a difference between being political and being partial. An evaluator needs to be politically aware, but also disinterested and not biased towards any party.

Access and co-operation

It is always difficult to get access to the data you will need. In many evaluations in developing countries it is advisable to visit the village or tribal chief before gathering data. This is paying respect to people and to the culture. It is also necessary for gaining the co-operation of many members of the community. There are similar rituals in developed countries.

Politics and motives can affect how easy it is for the evaluator to get access to and co-operation from personnel and patients. The evaluator will need access to documentation and statistics and to service providers to interview them. Access involves getting the formal agreement of the service manager, but getting helpful co-operation is more difficult and more important. The evaluator must be seen as someone who understands the practical problems and work situation of people in the service and is prepared to be flexible in scheduling interviews and visits. They also need to be seen as persistent and as someone who stands up to those from whom co-operation is required but who see the evaluation as low priority or who have something to hide.

A trusted, fair professional who 'speaks our language' is a model which an evaluator might aim for. Evaluators need to be aware of their 'image' on the informal work network or 'grapevine'; in small organisations a new face is an important event and myths and explanations of who the person is and their background will be rife and will affect access and co-operation. Fantasies will flower when the newcomer is known to be doing an evaluation. Co-operation can be damaged if the evaluator has not prepared the ground by being introduced in the right way and by meeting and showing respect for formal and informal opinion formers and different representatives.

Co-operation is increased if the evaluator gives something back to those whose time and efforts have been given to the evaluation. This is also a matter of evaluation ethics, not just a technique to get co-operation. Discussions with sponsors and others at the planning stage need to consider how service personnel and patients will benefit from the evaluation whilst it is being carried out, as well as after, and their contribution and role need to be acknowledged. This can take the form of interim reports, but this is not possible in summative evaluations where evaluator-influenced change is to be minimised. Texts giving practical guidance for evaluation and for health service research also discuss how to 'negotiate access' and present and introduce the evaluation to an organisation (e.g. Rossi and Freeman (1993), Fink (1993), Breakwell and Millward (1995)).

Credibility and trust

Establishing trust and credibility is essential to a successful evaluation. Following ethical evaluation practice helps to establish and maintain trust and professionalism. Trust and credibility have to be earned by the evaluator and will be tested. Both are required in the evaluator's relation-ships with different parties, most notably with sponsors, users, service personnel and patients. Everyone will want to find out from the evaluator what has been learned so far and to hear the latest 'inside' information, especially where organisational communications are poor. The more confidential the information, the more interested people will be, the faster it will be spread across the organisation if the evaluator breaks confidence and the quicker the evaluator's credibility will be lost.

Trust takes time to establish and is a result of the evaluator balancing honesty and discretion. Credibility comes from proving one's compet-ence but also from pointing out the limits to this competence. The proposal stage is where aspiring evaluators have to prove both their scientific and social competence by paying attention to and understand-ing sponsors' and users' concerns, being flexible, giving alternative designs and in the more conventional ways by showing their previous work and experience. Evaluators win trust by being cautious in their promises and by honestly answering and predicting questions about finance, possible problems and the limits to their skills and resources.

To gain access to an organisation, personnel and data, an evaluator has to spend some time preparing the ground and introducing themselves. These introductory activities are especially important for gaining trust. Researchers are often not welcome because they 'get in the way' and 'create extra work' and are often treated with suspicion. 'So, you have come to spy on us?' is not an uncommon welcome when being introduced and it is not always a joking question. Evaluation is not a neutral activity, even if the idea of being a neutral scientist is important to many evaluators. It helps to be introduced by a respected member of the organisation, but the evaluator must be prepared for and directly and honestly answer challenging questions, such as those which imply that the evaluation is not needed because a decision has already been made.

Confidentiality

A necessary precondition for gaining and maintaining access, co-operation and trust is to agree and make explicit how the information gathered will be reported and made available, even if people do not ask. When negotiating access to patient records and service documents which are not public, the evaluator needs to agree with service providers which information can and cannot be reported to sponsors and users or published (Øvretveit, 1986). This needs to be discussed at the planning stage with sponsors, as restrictions on access to and use of service records limit the data which can be gathered and shape the evaluation design. The evaluator should not discover part way into an evaluation that they cannot access essential data. These conditions and agreements need to be written down in the evaluation contract.

Confidentiality issues also arise when interviewing patients, service personnel and others. All interviews need to begin with the evaluator stating their understanding of the confidentiality rules which apply to the interview. Often it is best to give the interviewee a written statement of these conditions beforehand, together with a general explanation of the evaluation. The conditions need to state whether anything said in the interview will be attributed to the individual in a report or repeated outside the interview. One approach is for the evaluator to say that no individuals will be named or recognisable from the report and that only general findings will be reported when they have been supported by evidence from more than one source.

Evaluators also need to state any circumstances under which their code of ethical practice requires them to break confidentiality, which is often the code of their 'home profession'. Some service providers feel that their only chance to report corruption, abuse, negligence or other activities is to the evaluator. Evaluators need to know what the usual channels are within the organisation for dealing with such reports and to decide and agree beforehand how to respond in these circumstances. Even with foresight, evaluators may be faced with weighing up how to act to cause the least harm and to uphold their integrity, even if this means jeopardising the whole evaluation.

The questions of the public or private status of the final evaluation report and of publication rights should also be agreed with sponsor and service providers at the beginning of the evaluation. Many people will want to know what the evaluator found out and the evaluator needs to agree who will make their report available and what they can and cannot say in public and in informal settings during and after the evaluation.

The evaluation contract

Evaluators and sponsors can prevent many problems and misunderstandings by drawing up a contract which defines responsibilities and agreements about many of the items above. A good evaluation proposal should cover many of the above items in the design or in a separate heading about 'practical issues'. The proposal can serve as the contract or additions can be made in a separate contract agreement. There are different views about whether the evaluator should draw up contracts with other parties in addition to the financial sponsor. In many cases a clear contract which describes responsibilities and expectations can enhance trust, rather than suggesting mistrust.

Communicating evaluation findings

Communicating with many different types of people is an important ability for an evaluator and communicating findings is one of the phases of an evaluation. Here we consider the evaluator's responsibility for communicating their findings and the different ways in which they can do so.

Communication happens when the 'receiver' understands what the 'sender' intended to convey. Dialogue is a two-way exchange where both reach a new level of understanding. Dialogue is essential in the early phases of an evaluation to agree criteria, but communication is where the emphasis lies for the evaluator when reporting their findings.

A well-designed and conducted evaluation is wasted if users do not understand the findings and their limitations and significance. An evaluation can be harmful if users misunderstand the findings. It is arguable that the evaluator has a greater ethical duty than other researchers to clearly communicate their findings. Evaluations can have an immediate impact on people's lives and misunderstandings about the findings can have serious economic, social or health consequences.

Many users and evaluators agree that evaluators are often ill equipped to make recommendations for action, in part because they often do not know all the factors which users have to consider. However, evaluators do have a duty to go beyond putting a report in the mail to the sponsor or giving a simple presentation and then leaving. They have a duty to check that users have understood what the evaluation does and does not prove, but also a duty to resist being drawn into advising users about what they should do.

> *Those who stand to lose from an evaluation are not as crude as to shoot the messenger – they just destroy the credibility of the message.*

There are a number of ways to communicate findings to users: a verbal presentation or presentations at conferences; a workshop; a written report specifically for users or published in a 'users' journal'; putting the findings on a database or dissemination network which is accessed by users; informal discussions; and a press event such as a press release, a newspaper interview or a radio or television appearance. The most common ways are written or verbal presentations, but before the evaluator decides to use these methods they need to think about exactly who their audience is and what is the best way to communicate findings to them. Apart from the sponsor and other users agreed at the outset, the evaluation may have made discoveries which need to be communicated to other users such as patients. An evaluator may only be familiar with communicating to researchers or academics and may need advice or help to communicate the findings to users or to hand over the communication to specialists.

Most general and practical texts on research give guidance about how to write a report, but most of this guidance is for an academic report or a scientific paper for publication. Writing a report for non-academic users such as health managers, practitioners, policy makers and the general public often follows similar principles and headings, but does require a different style and approach. For health evaluators reporting to health personnel, more useful guidance is given in two texts specifically for evaluators: Breakwell and Millward (1995, Chapter 6) and Fink (1993, Chapter 8).

Ethical evaluation

Do no harm.

The time to worry about ethics is when you think there are no ethical issues.

Evaluation is not just following professional technical methods: these will not help in many situations and technique is often blind to the ethical issues. Evaluator ethics protect the weak and minimises the harm to different parties which can result from an unskilful evaluation. This is the main reason for carrying out an evaluation in an ethical way – to avoid harming people, especially the powerless and vulnerable, and to maximise the good which comes from your work. Another reason is because ethical principles also help to improve the technical quality of an evaluation, especially in situations where there is no technical guidance. For example, a patient or health professional may report a serious abuse to the evaluator. Not dealing with this issue in an ethical way will damage the evaluator's credibility and their access to data in the future.

Many of the ethical aspects of carrying out an evaluation were discussed in the last section. We saw that evaluation should make a difference and that different groups will win or lose from the evaluation or will perceive themselves as so doing. Evaluations have a great potential for doing harm. I have known hurriedly undertaken evaluations which have destroyed the work of many years. One report was used to close a project when the evaluator had not interviewed any beneficiaries of the programme or taken into account the changing and difficult conditions under which the project had been operating.

The discussion above drew attention to the political issues and to practical ways through the minefield. Evaluation ethics also give practical guidance but are based more on principles than pragmatism. They are principles which also help to minimise predictable problems and to enhance the validity of the evaluation. In a discussion of the ethics of evaluation, House (1980) describes five ethical mistakes.

- *Clientism*: doing whatever the customer wants
- *Managerialism*: seeing managers as the only users
- *Methodologicalism*: assuming that following the technically correct methods is the same as being ethical
- *Relativism*: that all opinions are of equal value
- *Elitism*: giving the most powerful the strongest voice.

An ethical approach to evaluation includes being aware of the choices you make as an evaluator, of the consequences of these choices for different parties and of using ethical principles in making these choices. We have seen the choices the evaluator faces about evaluation design and data-gathering methods and choices to be made in different phases of the evaluation. These choices have consequences for the people providing the programme or implementing the change, the most obvious being that some choices mean using up more of their time than others. Awareness of the impact ranges from recognising that interviewing health personnel or asking for data takes their time away from patient care to being aware how the phrasing of a key part of a report may be used to justify cutting funding for a programme or could lead to a person losing their job.

It is often difficult to predict the consequences of the choices which the evaluator makes. It is also not the responsibility of the evaluator to step ouside the limits of the evaluation and influence decisions which should be made by users or which should be political decisions. There is a fine line between an ethical approach and a political approach. This is why the stress is on awareness of choices and consequences.

In my experience the two most important ethical injunctions to remember in the busyness of the evaluation process are: do no harm, and start worrying about the ethics of what you are doing if you think there are no ethical issues. Some of the main ethical principles to guide choice of action in an evaluation are:

- treating others as you would have them treat you or as if everyone should act in this way (universalist)
- treating people equally (one principle of justice)
- treating people with different needs unequally (fairness)
- acting so that the least well off are made better off (another principle of justice)
- acting to achieve the greatest happiness for the greatest number or to achieve the greatest benefit for the least cost (utilitarian)
- acting in ways which respect and do not violate other people's wishes and feelings (respect)
- recognising the unique and equal value of every living person (absolutist, or natural rights)
- acting in a way which develops the spiritual awareness of ourselves and others (spiritual).

An ethical approach does not just mean acting on a principle, it means considering alternatives before deciding which principle is the most important. Indeed, it could be argued that the over-riding principle is the need to search for the principle which is most important to observe in the situation. An ethical approach means being aware of values, one's own and those of other people, because values help to decide which is the most important principle in the situation.

Deciding which value criteria to use to assess an intervention is where awareness of your own and others' values is important. We saw in a discussion of value criteria in Chapter 6 that a user-focused approach does not mean ignoring values other than those of the users. The evaluator's ethics and values may lead them to suggest value criteria which have not been considered, such as equity or justice for the poor. But how far should the evaluator's ethics and values enter into the evaluation? One view is that:

> *Evaluation cannot simply concern itself with the success or otherwise of the initiative, but must try to answer ethical, political, philosophical and social questions about the good life with particular reference to health.* (Scott and Weston, 1998)

An ethical evaluator will give a high priority to the communication phase because sponsors have paid for users to become more informed, not just paid for an evaluation to be conducted. The evaluator has a duty clearly to communicate their findings and to assist in exploring the implications. They have a duty to go to some lengths to ensure that users do not misinterpret the results. They need to know when and how to resist pressures to give advice about action. In communicating evaluation results, it is wise to assume that everything will be misheard or misread and that the report will only be studiously scrutinised by those who disagree with the results.

Deciding what to do in carrying out an evaluation is difficult because:

- we have a choice
- we do not know the consequences of the choice for other people
- acting in one way will benefit one person or group, but harm or disbenefit another
- whatever we do will go against one or more ethical principles.

There would be no need of ethics in evaluation if:

- there were no imbalances of power
- there were laws and rules to follow for each situation, which prevented the misuse of power and promoted 'good' acts
- we think that there are no choices: ethics operates in the space left by the laws and regulations and in deciding how to apply the laws.

Evaluation ethics anticipate many of the practical challenges discussed earlier in this and the other chapters: ethical evaluation practice is not just something evaluators strive for in order to sleep easy at night, but something which enhances the validity of the findings and is essential to the future reputation of evaluation as a practice and as a discipline.

For more discussion of ethics the reader is referred to Newman and Brown (1998), the detailed codes for US programme evaluation (JCSEE, 1994) and Menckel and Westerholm (1999), as well as to codes specifically for medical research and to Scott and Weston (1998) for a discussion of ethics in health promotion.

Summary

- Evaluators need to understand how the interests of different groups could be affected by an evaluation in order to plan and conduct their evaluation and to increase the chances of their work being acted on. They need to be 'streetwise'.
- Political awareness is important to understand unacknowledged agendas and motives for carrying out an evaluation, how to get access and co-operation, how to build credibility and trust, confidentiality and how to communicate evaluation findings
- Evaluator ethics minimise the harm to different parties which can result from an unskilful evaluation.

- Ethics are principles which help to minimise predictable problems and to enhance the validity of the evaluation.
- An ethical approach includes being aware of the choices and of the consequences of the choices you make as an evaluator and using ethical principles in making these choices.
- An ethical approach is not without conflict: following one ethical principle usually means going against another principle and, at worst, hurting some people. The question is, which is the over-riding ethical principle to try to follow in the situation?

Chapter 13

Evaluating quality and qualefficiency

'Quality evaluation' can mean many things: measuring quality, comparing levels of quality, assessing a quality system or programme or research into the cause of poor quality.

The level of quality provided by a service depends on the resources available. Qualefficiency evaluation assesses the quality achieved for the resources available and focuses attention on actions which both reduce costs and improve quality at the same time

Introduction

Most managers and professionals are required to carry out quality evaluation, by law or as a contractual or professional duty. Quality evaluation is necessary for quality improvement, but there are questions about which methods are the most effective. Are the benefits of the many types of quality inspections and evaluations worth the costs? There is much duplication and uncertainty about who should be carrying out different quality activities. There is also a tension between the methods of inspection which are favoured by governments to ensure that basic standards are met and developmental methods which encourage self-improvement. Quality evaluation is now everyone's business, but it is not always clear which methods to use or which are the most cost-effective and there is a need to evaluate the many methods which are used.

Evaluation is political and so is quality. Different interest groups support definitions of quality and evaluation methods which defend and advance their interests. This in part explains some of the confusion of terms. Any definition or specification of quality is a value judgement, a choice to focus on some things and exclude others. The act of collecting data about quality performance is threatening for many and can give information which allows greater control over organisations and clinicians. Put quality and evaluation together and the practical and technical challenges increase for the evaluator, as we will see in this chapter.

Quality and evaluation are closely linked. There is an increasing overlap and inter-relation between different activities.

- Many services themselves carry out quality measurement and evaluation as a part of their own quality activities. If the measurement methods they use are standardised then comparisons can be made between services.
- Evaluators are sometimes asked to evaluate both the quality of a service and the quality system which a service is using at one time to ensure its quality. They may also be asked to evaluate the service's quality programme or strategy which ranges over a period of time.
- Services use reported evaluations to improve quality; for example, professionals use research evaluations to formulate guidelines and managers use research into other successful or failed quality programmes.

'Quality evaluation' has become a general term for a wide range of activities. The subject is confusing because people use the words 'quality' and 'evaluation' to mean different things. After reading this chapter you will be able to:

- describe the five types of 'quality evaluation', their different purposes and methods (Box 13.1)
- explain why quality evaluations are required and for whom they are carried out
- follow a series of steps for carrying out an internal or external quality evaluation
- explain what 'qualefficiency' is and why assessing qualefficiency gives a fairer view of the performance of a health organisation.

Doctors, nurses and some managers know about an 'iron law of the universe'. That the quality achieved by a service is relative – relative to the number of people it serves, to the severity of their needs or illness and to the resources available. In the past most service quality evaluations were absolute and did not consider these factors. Evaluations and comparisons are beginning to take account of patient variables such as severity of illness, but not the resources available to a service.

There is a relationship between the quality of a service and the resources which people have available to provide the service. To make a fair evaluation we need to relate the level of quality to the resources as well as to the number and type of people served. The concept of 'qualefficiency' allows an evaluation of quality in relation to resources. Qualefficiency is using the fewest resources to achieve a consistent standard of care, which meets a defined number of patients' essential health needs and wants. The chapter later discusses this concept and shows how to measure qualefficiency to give a more integrated performance measure than that of quality alone.

Box 13.1: Five types of 'quality evaluation' – which type of quality evaluation is needed?

Type 1: a measurement of the quality of a service (a 'quality performance measurement')

Type 2: a judgement of the value of the quality performance of a service, compared with its performance one year ago or with the performance of a similar service at the same time (a 'service quality evaluation')

Type 3: an inspection of the arrangements a service has at one time for ensuring quality (an 'evaluation of a quality system')

Type 4: an assessment of a quality programme of different activities and structures introduced to train, motivate and support personnel to ensure and improve quality (an 'evaluation of a quality programme')

Type 5: a research study to understand the causes of high or low quality performance (a 'research quality evaluation')

Why evaluate quality?

The choice of which type of quality evaluation to carry out depends on the evaluation user's needs. The purpose of a quality evaluation is to help someone to act differently or to make a more informed decision than they would otherwise do without the evaluation findings. Different people can use the results of a quality evaluation. Who might want a quality evaluation and for which purposes?

To inform and assure patients

In the past patients or patient associations rarely asked for or sponsored service quality evaluations, but this is changing. Patients now want independent quality evaluations – they are less trusting that professionals always put patients' needs first or that a public service will assure quality. Patients want the work of professionals to be judged according to patients' criteria of value, as well as according to professional criteria. Sometimes the motive is an accident or instance of poor care. Patients want to know if the instance is more general or could happen again and want to judge whether it could happen to them before they undergo care. Examples are neglect in care homes for older people, poor after-care or questionable deaths after surgery, all of which may move patients to call for a quality evaluation. Other motives are that patients want information about quality in order to be able to make an informed choice of provider.

To protect the voiceless and uphold equity

Another reason to assess quality is that some patients or clients are less able to express their views. The views of people with dementia, very disabled people and homeless people are often ignored, but they have equal rights and should be treated as equal human beings. There are many patients who rarely make their views about quality heard to service providers or to others. Service providers often do not have the time, expertise or incentives to find out how people without power or a voice value their service.

In public services, quality evaluations are even more necessary than other types of evaluation for upholding social values of equity. Articulate and well-organised educated groups are more able to get resources diverted to meet their needs, at the expense of others who do not lobby so hard. Managers and others need to know how less powerful people value the service in order to act in their interests and counter the pressures of the vocal groups. Evaluations can use techniques to find out how people value a service when these people have difficulty or are reluctant to express their views (JRF, 2001). It is all too easy for evaluators and others to impose their own criteria rather than eliciting and using those of such patients, at least as one set of criteria in the evaluation. We need to ask, who sponsors and initiates quality evaluations for the voiceless and disempowered?

For professional purposes

Professionals are a second interest group which want service quality evaluations and for a number of purposes. First, professional pride and professional vocation. Most professions declare that a duty of their members is to evaluate their own practice and to take part in evaluations to improve services and maintain standards. This in turn derives from professionals' espoused principle of 'service' and their intention to put the interests of patients above all others. Many professions themselves run quality evaluation programmes for their members and have done so for many years. More recently, other reasons have led professionals to be involved in quality evaluations. In many countries there is now a requirement that professionals take part in quality assurance or co-operate with external quality evaluations; for example, recent laws passed in Norway and Sweden. A further reason is that evaluating quality helps professionals to monitor the impact of cuts to finance or changes in a service on the quality of their service. Generally, the purpose of evaluating quality from the professional perspective is self-improvement and this can be carried out through either self-evaluation or external evaluation.

For management purposes

A third set of reasons for evaluating quality comes from the management perspective and from health managers at different levels. There are three answers to the question 'why evaluate quality?' from this group. The first is that managers are responsible for ensuring that tax-payers' money is well spent. If they pay attention only to the more easily measured costs and quantity of services, they will miss the third corner of the 'value-for-money triangle' of cost–quantity–quality. The second reason is that health managers have a responsibility to all of the population served by a service, not just those 'passing through' it. They need to assess the service's availability to all the population and some definitions of quality include these more comprehensive features of a service ('population quality'; Øvretveit, 1999). The third reason is more political and rarely stated – to increase managers' power over and control of professionals, who claim exclusive ability to assess and regulate their own quality. Independent quality evaluation can provide management with credible data to justify their plans.

This third set of management reasons overlaps with those of government. In addition to ensuring value for money, governments have a duty to protect citizens from harm which may come from citizens' inability to assess professional quality – this applies to any service. Governments have additional responsibilities as owners and providers of public services to reduce unacceptable or preventable risks for patients and service personnel.

A final reason for evaluating health service quality is to contribute to scientific knowledge, rather than to any immediate and direct practical purpose. Little is known about the relationships between outcome and processes and the methods of evaluation have much to contribute to understanding the causes of high and low quality outcomes from systems of care.

Box 13.2: Why evaluate quality?

- For patients to be able to make informed choices about which service to use or whether to undergo a treatment.
- To ensure that the quality judgements of people who have little power or voice are recognised.
- For professionals to improve their practice and monitor the effects of service changes on their quality of practice.
- For managers to assess value for money, ensure all patients' interests are served and increase control over professionals.
- For governments to protect the public.
- To contribute to scientific knowledge about the causes of high and low quality outcomes from systems of care.

Defining and measuring quality

Defining quality is a precondition for measuring it. Measuring quality itself is of no value unless the measures are used to compare one service's quality performance with others or with itself at an earlier time – to evaluate quality. They are also used in quality improvement projects to identify problems and solutions and to evaluate the effects of changes. Later we look at evaluation; here we consider definitions of quality and how these definitions help us to focus on what to measure.

Which aspects of the service does the evaluator assess? A general answer is those aspects of quality which are important to the users of the evaluation. These are the value criteria to be used in the evaluation and against which the service is to be judged. Sometimes these criteria can be specified by the evaluation users, for example by professionals or managers who are concerned about whether quality standards are met or regulations are followed by personnel. Sometimes work needs to be done with service users to specify the value criteria which they use (e.g. symptom relief, treated with dignity). Sometimes the evaluator can use definitions and specifications of quality which others have developed (e.g. the King's Fund organisational audit; Brooks, 1992). Often evaluators draw on all three to specify the value criteria, before moving on to decide how to gather data about how the service performs in relation to these value criteria.

Definitions of service quality for evaluation purposes

Quality assurance is a discipline which has created many different definitions of quality which can be used to decide operational measures of quality. These definitions can be used in discussions with evaluation users to agree which aspect of the service to evaluate. One 'dimensional' definition of quality which is helpful for deriving criteria for a quality evaluation is that of Maxwell (1984), who defines the following dimensions:

- *accessibility*: distance, time, social barriers
- *relevance to need*: 'appropriateness'
- *equity*: equal services for equal needs, unequal services for unequal needs
- *social acceptability*: that what is provided and the manner in which it is provided are acceptable
- *effectiveness*: produces the desired effect in everyday conditions
- *efficiency*: for example, produces the desired effect with the least waste, such as at a low cost and in an economical way.

Maxwell's definition is comprehensive (too broad for some purposes) and covers areas of interest to different evaluation users. It is useful for defining the quality of purchasing and is similar to that of the Joint Commission for Accreditation of Healthcare Organisations (JCAHO), which adds 'continuity', gives a different emphasis to some of the dimensions and links them.

- *Efficacy*: is the treatment useful?
- *Appropriateness*: is it right for this patient?
- *Accessibility*: if it is right, can the patient get it?
- *Effectiveness*: is it carried out well?
- *Efficiency*: is it carried out in a cost-effective way?
- *Continuity*: did the treatment progress without interruption, with appropriate follow-up, exchange of information and referral?

However, in both these definitions the usual emphasis on quality as patient satisfaction has been lost. It is also debatable whether a definition captures the holistic nature of quality: our perception of quality is not the sum total of its elements – the elements combine to give a perception which is greater than the sum of the elements. This 'system' feature of the perception of quality is also a feature of how quality is created: quality assurance and quality programmes can ensure linkage between quality activities to create an impact which is more than the sum of the activities. This is an important aspect of quality to bear in mind in a quality evaluation and something which dimensional or reductionist definitions rarely capture.

A general definition of the quality of a service is whether it 'meets the health needs of those most in need at the lowest cost, and within regulations' (Øvretveit, 1992a). This definition can be used to assess a service from three perspectives as it involves the three dimensions of:

1 *Patient quality*: whether the service gives patients what they want
2 *Professional quality*: professionals' views of whether the service meets patients' needs as assessed by professionals (outcome being one measure) and whether staff correctly select and carry out procedures which are believed to be necessary to meeting patients' needs (process)
3 *Management quality*: the most efficient and productive use of resources to meet client needs, without waste and within limits and directives set by higher authorities.

Donabedian's conceptualisation of structure, process and outcome (Donabedian, 1980) is not a definition of quality as such but it can be usefully combined with other definitions to give a framework for measuring quality (Table 13.1). Another useful framework for identifying ways to measure quality is to draw a patient pathway diagram and measure quality at different points on the patient's path through the service (a process-based measurement system discussed in Øvretveit (1992a, b, 1993), Nelson *et al.*, 1996) and Nelson and Batalden, 1993).

This framework can be used to identify which measures of quality to use in a service quality evaluation (based on Donabedian, 1980, and Øvretveit, 1992a, b).

Which definition the evaluator uses depends on the purpose of the evaluation and who it is for. Some definitions are more suited to primary healthcare services, some to primary services with a range of social and other services, some to complex secondary or tertiary specialist care services, some to support or diagnostic services and some to evaluating the quality of purchasing or financing organisations. An evaluator needs

Table 13.1: Quality measurement framework

	Input The right amount and quality of:	Process Activities of care	Outcomes Change in patient's experience, health and resources that can be attributed to the service's actions
Patient quality What patients say they want or what is necessary in inputs process or outcomes to give patients what they want	e.g. well-qualified and experienced health personnel Clean and attractive buildings and facilities.	e.g. polite and friendly treatment by health personnel The right amount of information at each stage of the treatment No unnecessary pain Quick service when required	e.g. patient satisfaction Pain reduction or elimination Return to activities
Professional quality Professionals' views about whether the service meets patients' needs, whether staff correctly select and carry out procedures which are believed to be necessary to meet patients' needs	e.g. well-trained and co-operative colleagues The right patients are referred Sufficient information about patients is provided The right equipment Access to efficient support services	e.g. correct diagnosis Correct choice of intervention Compliance with procedures Fast support services Good interprofessional communication	e.g. good health outcome No negative outcomes
Management quality The most efficient and productive use of resources to meet client needs within limits and directives set by higher authorities	e.g. sufficient resources Good external services and information	e.g. no waste, error or delays Compliance with higher level regulations	e.g. lowest costs per patient Fewest resources consumed

to be familiar with these and other definitions in order to help users who are not sure what they mean by quality to decide exactly what they want the evaluation to look for and for which purposes. More details about how to measure quality are given in Nelson *et al.* (1996), Nelson and Batalden (1993), Berwick *et al.* (1990), Blumenthal and Scheck (1995) and Øvretveit (1992a, b, 1993).

Box 13.3: A quality evaluation needs to:

- decide the *general definition of quality* (e.g. the ability of a service to satisfy patients or a wider definition)
- decide which *aspects to assess* (e.g. waiting time, pain control, qualifications of personnel – the value criteria)
- decide how to *operationalise* these aspects for data gathering or measurement (e.g. time recorded from registration to doctor recording time of arrival for consultation, patient's record of number of times they called for a nurse for pain relief, etc.)
- decide which *comparison* to use to judge the quality performance achieved on the measure (e.g. over time, or between services).

Evaluating service quality

Measuring quality is different from evaluating quality. Sometimes managers ask for a quality evaluation, meaning that they want someone to measure the quality of a service. They might not know which things to measure or might recognise the political issues involved and want someone else to define quality and measure it. Measurement involves making a value judgement to decide which things are important – for example, waiting times and a caring attitude. One approach is to find out what patients value and measure the service against these criteria. However, a single measurement of quality of itself is not very useful.

Evaluating quality usually involves measuring quality but more as well: making a judgement about the measured levels of quality performance and their significance. This valuation of the level of quality is made by comparing the measured quality of a service with its level previously or with a similar service. The purpose of doing this is to decide action; for example, should we keep the change we made to improve quality?

The quality of a service is how well it meets patients' needs and wants. We saw above that we need a more specific definition of quality to then decide how to measure it. Once the evaluator has decided which measures of quality to use, the question is, which type of comparison to use to judge the value of the quality performance achieved? The following shows common designs for service quality evaluations. Each uses a different type of comparison, apart from the first design.

Type 1: descriptive

This is a single case study design to describe the service inputs and activities which are relevant from a quality perspective. It is not a common design and not considered an evaluation by some. It can be used in an initial investigation to decide how to define the service and which aspects of quality to investigate further or concentrate on improving. The evaluator uses a quality theory to guide which aspects of the services they describe.

Type 2: audit

In this design the evaluator compares the service with standards or quality objectives and gives evidence of the extent to which the service meets the standards or objectives. An example is a medical or nursing audit of the treatment of a patient group compared to agreed standards or protocols or using an organisation audit or accreditation schedule (Brooks, 1992; Edgren, 1995; Øvretveit, 1994a). There are three types of audit designs.

- Type 2a: the evaluator uses quality standards which have already been formulated and applies them to audit the service.
- Type 2b: the evaluator develops the standards or criteria against which to audit the service, often in collaboration with the evaluation users.
- Type 2c: the evaluator takes the quality objectives defined by the service, decides how to operationalise these for data gathering and collects evidence of the extent to which the service achieved its own quality objectives. Quality objectives usually include quality standards.

Type 3: time comparison – single service

The comparison in this type of design is between the quality of the service at one time compared to another time. The simplest version of this design is a repeat audit, comparing how well the service met audit standards at time 1 with time 2. Another version of this design compares the same group of patients' assessments of the same service at different times. An example is a group of elderly people in a nursing home assessing the quality of the service at different times. A variation is a comparison of patients' expectations before receiving the services with the same patients' experiences after. An example is the SERVQUAL customer satisfaction measurement schedule applied in health services by Babakus and Mangold (1992). A further version of this design compares the assessment of different groups of patients. An example is measuring patient satisfaction of one group of patients and comparing this with the measured satisfaction of a similar group at a later time.

These designs are sometimes called 'trend evaluations'. They involve defining which aspects of quality to measure at different times. They are of most use to the service for quality improvement if the evaluator assesses aspects of quality which can be influenced by the service.

Type 4: service comparison

This design gathers data about the quality of two or more services and compares their quality performance. The design can compare patient satisfaction or other quality outcomes or how well two or more services meet standards. A version of this design is a combination of two or more type 3 comparisons. For example, the evaluation gathers data about patient satisfaction for each service separately, calculates for each service the difference or trend over time and then compares the trends across services, thus showing how much patient satisfaction has changed for each service. If the patient groups and other factors are similar for different services, this allows the evaluator to apply a degree of control for the factors other than the service which affect quality performance and make more valid comparisons between services.

Each design serves different purposes and is useful for answering different questions. Which design to use depends on the needs of the evaluation user, the resources available for the evaluation and the time constraints. It also depends on the skills and role of the evaluator: the evaluator may be internal to the service (clinicians or a manager) or external to the service (an inspector or accreditation agent or a researcher).

Evaluating a quality system or quality programme

There are a category of 'quality evaluations' which do not measure or evaluate the quality of service directly. These evaluate a quality system or a quality programme which an organisation uses to ensure and improve quality. There are three main types. The first is a 'research evaluation of a quality system'. Examples of such research are an evaluation of the DySSSy nursing quality system (Kitson *et al.*, 1994), an evaluation of the Swedish version of the King's Fund organisational audit system (Edgren, 1995) and a comparative evaluation of ISO-9000, King's Fund and Baldridge systems (including the European Quality Foundation Model) in healthcare (Øvretveit, 1994a).

The second is an assessment of whether a service has a system in place or how well a service is following a system. These latter types are often called system inspections, system audits or quality system accreditations. For example, Norway has a law requiring all health organisations to have a quality system and has government inspectors who check if the law is being followed (Sh, 1995). The inspector-evaluators do not measure quality directly but check that the service uses an approved system. For other countries considering such an approach, one of the lessons from the Norwegian experience is that guidance is needed about which systems are most effective for particular organisations in different circumstances. Such guidance should ideally be based on research evaluations of quality systems.

The third type is an evaluation of a quality programme which an organisation introduces to improve quality such as a total quality management programme. Quality programmes usually involve different activities such as a training programme, quality projects, a quality project management process and may also include a programme to introduce a quality system. Evaluations of a quality programme can be carried out as an internal review or by an external evaluator as a research evaluation. Examples of the latter are evaluations of the NHS TQM programme (Joss and Kogan, 1995), of TQM programmes in primary healthcare (Lawrence and Packwood, 1996) and of the quality programmes of six Norwegian hospitals (Øvretveit, 1999).

Designs for evaluating a hospital quality programme

There are six main designs for evaluating a hospital quality programme (Øvretveit, 1997). A quality programme is an 'intentional change' to an organisation. The targets of this intervention are hospital personnel and organisation, not patients, although improvement in patient care is an intended long-term outcome.

The first design is a case study evaluation to describe the programme and its history. The features to be described would depend on the evaluation user's questions and criteria of valuation. One management question is, what is the value of the programme to health service personnel and what do we need to do to increase people's motivation to work on quality improvement?

A second design is to study the service providers who are the target of the programme and ask them what they think of the programme, its progress and impact (the main method used by Lawrence and Packwood, 1996). A third approach is to take the service's quality plan and objectives and compare these to what had actually been done in the service. A drawback is that a service may not define the objectives of the programme or describe them only in general way. The latter requires the evaluator to specify how to measure the attainment of objectives, ideally in collaboration with those who devised the programme. Showing the lack of evaluatable plans and objectives can itself help to develop the programme.

A fourth approach is to compare what the service has done with a prescriptive model of what a service should do to pursue a successful quality programme. There is no lack of such prescriptions in the quality literature, but not many are suitable for public health services and most also emphasise the importance of adapting the model to a particular service. One option is for the evaluator to develop their own model by drawing on the quality literature (e.g. Joss and Kogan, 1995; Øvretveit and Aslaksen, 1999).

A fifth approach is to measure directly the quality of the service before and at different intervals during the quality programme. In theory this is what the service should itself do and it may be possible to draw on measures collected by the service as well as making independent direct measures. In practice few services have measures of quality before they started the programme; it is common for an evaluation to be requested some time after the programme has been running. A sixth approach is to use a framework of key choices which all services face when pursuing a quality programme and compare the service's choices to those of other services. More details about methods for internal and external evaluations of quality programmes in health services are discussed in Joss *et al.* (1994), Joss and Kogan (1995) and Øvretveit (1997, 1999).

Table 13.2: Types of quality evaluation

	Carried out by internal evaluator		Carried out by external evaluator	
	Caregivers	Management	Inspector	Researcher
1 Measurement	Often	Often	Rarely	Rarely
2 Service quality evaluation	Often	Often	Sometimes	Sometimes
3 Evaluation of a quality system	Sometimes	Sometimes	Often	Sometimes
4 Evaluation of a quality programme	Never	Sometimes	Never	Sometimes
5 Research evaluation of causes of quality	Sometimes, in a quality project	Never	Never	Sometimes

Evaluating qualefficiency: an integrated approach to performance assessment

Qualefficiency is using the fewest resources to achieve a consistent standard of care, which meets a defined number of patients' essential health needs and wants.

Similar designs and methods to those described above can be used to evaluate qualefficiency. The following explains this concept and how it can be measured as part of a qualefficiency evaluation.

The level of quality achieved by a service depends on many factors, one of which is the resources available. If we use a measure which combines quality and efficiency then we can make better comparisons between services or between one service over time: the measure allows us to take account of resource differences. We can also see whether a service is using quality methods effectively to reduce costs and improve quality at the same time. This is why the qualefficiency concept brings together quality, efficiency and effectiveness to define the resources needed to achieve a standard of care which meets a certain number of patients' essential health requirements.

The concept focuses attention on the most important performance aspects of health organisations. Evaluating qualefficiency gives management and health professionals the information which they need to prioritise improvements and to assess whether resources are being allocated in the best way.

Why not assess quality and then separately assess other aspects of the performance of a health organisation? One reason is that quality and other aspects of performance need to be considered together, in an integrated performance measure. Another is that changes in recent years have led to a convergence of methods and concerns about quality, costs and effectiveness. Governments and health managers in the 1990s were preoccupied with increasing efficiency to reduce costs and contain healthcare expenditure. Evidence-based healthcare entered the picture in the mid-1990s, with its focus on effectiveness, and was viewed by some as a way of avoiding rationing. If public finance was only spent on treatments which were proven to be effective, then there may be enough public money to pay for all necessary healthcare.

At the same time the 1990s saw the rise of the quality movement which for many years flowed in parallel to the efficiency and effectiveness trends. For some reason many in public healthcare did not accept that quality methods could be used to reduce costs. Yet in the USA a change occurred in the mid-1990s with payers' resistance to rising healthcare costs. Quality methods were increasingly used to reduce costs. The 'improvement movement' represented the third phase of quality in healthcare, after the first profession-based approach and the second quality assurance approach. The improvement movement caught on in the USA because it provided a way of uniting professionals' concerns about quality with health funders' and managers' concerns about costs.

This lead to the current convergence of quality improvement, evidence-based healthcare and cost performance improvement, which is represented in the concept of qualefficiency. In public healthcare there has been little recognition that quality methods are for reducing errors and costs as well as for improving clinical and consumer quality. Qualefficiency development brings together techniques from the quality and evidence-based medicine movement with performance improvement methods to create high-quality and low-resource utilisation services.

> *The concept 'bridging' quality and efficiency is waste. Quality methods can reduce waste. Waste is activities which do not efficiently meet another person's need, where there is a known way to do so or one could be created at a low cost.*

Measuring qualefficiency

In order to evaluate qualefficiency we need to measure it and to measure it we need to define it in a way which points towards which measures we could use. The following gives one definition of three dimensions of qualefficiency.

1 *Patient qualefficiency*: the extent to which the service provides the level of service expected by a specified number of patients for the resources available.
2 *Professional qualefficiency*: the extent to which the service meets a specified number of patients' professionally defined needs which can be met with the resources available and uses methods which are thought to be able to meet this number of patients' needs and which are appropriate for the resources available.
3 *Management qualefficiency*: using the fewest resources to:
   • meet the required patient and professional quality standards, for the specified number of patients, without waste, delays and errors
   • operate an effective system to prevent errors and continuously improve patient and professional quality
   • comply with higher level regulations.

These definitions can be used to decide which specific measures to use. Examples are:

- patient satisfaction score/resources used for each patient (or cost per patient)
- professional quality measure (e.g. infection rates)/resources used for each patient (or cost per patient)
- the current 'cost of quality' calculated for a particular service (Øvretveit, 1991b, 2000b).

Once the specific measures of qualefficiency are fixed, the evaluator can then decide how to use these measures to evaluate qualefficiency. One way is to gather measures for a service at one time and compare these with the same measures one year later to see any changes. Another way is to compare two services at the same time. These comparisons make it possible to judge the value of the qualefficiency performance and also to track the effect of changes, such as a new IT system or a organisational restructuring.

Box 13.4: Myths about qualefficiency

- You cannot treat more patients for the same cost without lowering quality: there is an unchangeable relation between volume, cost and quality.
- Doctors, nurses and other disciplines will not co-operate in project teams to raise patient satisfaction, improve clinical outcomes and reduce costs at the same time.
- It is difficult to get doctors to lead qualefficiency programmes and to involve them in such strategies.
- Managers are not interested in clinical outcomes, only in reducing costs.
- Collecting data about quality, waste and efficiency is expensive and not worth the time and costs.

(The evidence is that services have used quality methods successfully to reduce waste and errors and at the same time improve clinical outcomes and patient satisfaction.)

Practical steps for a quality evaluation

Defining what is to be evaluated

'What do they want evaluated?' seemed a simple question to answer: an evaluation of the quality of primary healthcare centre. But the more we planned the evaluation, the more we questioned what should be included as part of the primary healthcare centre. The services provided by all full-time personnel at the centre? What about the work done at the centre by a visiting therapist one day a month? Is it to exclude the clinics which the centre's nurses run at another primary healthcare centre?

To evaluate something it is necessary to 'draw a boundary' around the item to be evaluated and to exclude other things which are not to be evaluated. It is usually more difficult to define a service or a programme than to define a treatment. Creating the definition involves describing the service components and preferably agreeing this description with the users and the service providers. In the case of an evaluation of a quality programme, it involves describing the components of the programme and ruling out those activities which will not be viewed as part of the programme. This can be difficult, especially in evaluations of national or regional quality programmes. One way to limit the scope of the evaluation is to use a time perspective to separate phases of a programme and to define some activities as the short-term outcomes of the initial activities of the programme.

To decide where to 'draw the boundary' it helps to have an understanding of which future actions are to be informed by the evaluation. The question 'Why do they want the evaluation?' helps the users and the evaluators to limit the study to those things which will help to make better decisions in the future. The next section in this chapter discusses the different users of a quality evaluation and their actions which the evaluation could inform. Quality evaluations always rapidly expand to cover many interesting aspects, but they need to be limited to the essential to be useful. This means asking 'What are the questions which users have and the decisions, choices and actions which users face in the future?' Examples are: Should I use this service? Should we invest more money in improving quality? Is this service complying with the higher level requirements for quality? Understanding when the results of the evaluation are required also helps to limit the study; more detailed or valid findings usually take longer but may be wasted if they are not available by the time important decisions are to be made.

Practical steps

When designing a quality evaluation there are five main considerations. The first is for whom the evaluation is to be carried out and the valuation criteria which they and the evaluator agree. The evaluation users may be practitioners who evaluate their own practice or a service as part of their self-improvement process (which may also be in response to an external requirement that they do so). Evaluation users may also be patients or patients associations, local or central government, service managers or purchasers. Often there are multiple users, which may mean that the evaluator has to prioritise between primary and secondary evaluation users to plan an achievable design.

The second consideration is whether the evaluation users have already defined criteria. If not, then the evaluator can work with them to develop criteria by showing them examples of quality criteria which may be suitable for the evaluation (e.g. organisational audit criteria (Brooks, 1992)) or different definitions of quality (e.g. patient, professional and management quality). The third consideration is whether the evaluation is to study the quality of the service or of a system or programme used by the service to assess quality. The fourth consideration is whether it is to be a special single evaluation, for example for management users to help them to design a quality programme, or whether it is to help set up a routine quality evaluation to be repeated, for example every year. If the latter, is the purpose of the evaluation to test different systems which could be used by the service to do their own routine quality evaluation? The fifth factor is, who carries out the evaluation? Is it to be an external evaluator independent of the organisation or an internal evaluator?

The following is an outline of steps which are suitable for a formal external single evaluation of service quality, where there are no pre-defined criteria.

Steps in evaluating quality

1 Clarify who the evaluation is for: who is asking for and/or paying for the evaluation and who will be the main users of the findings?
2 Clarify the decisions and action which could follow from the evaluation: what do they want the evaluation for?
3 Clarify evaluation criteria: how do they define and judge quality, which other perspectives do they want included, which perspectives does the evaluator think should be included and what then are the criteria of valuation of quality?

4 Define the item to be evaluated (e.g. service or quality system), the questions to be answered and the purpose of the evaluation.
5 Design and plan the quality evaluation.
6 Collect data which will allow users to judge the quality of the service.
7 Analyse and report findings which allow users to judge quality and to make better informed decisions.

Summary

- More quality evaluation is being undertaken in health services as a result of the growth of consumerism, government requirements, purchaser demands and the quality movement.
- Quality evaluation is confusing, contentious and a political subject and this adds to the technical difficulties in carrying out and using a quality evaluation. It is the task of the evaluator to be clear and explicit about the terms and purposes, not to compound the confusion or become an unwitting ally to a particular interest group.
- The difficulties can be reduced by being clear about who the evaluation is being done for and which decisions it should inform and knowing about the different methods for quality evaluation.
- Part of the confusion is because 'quality evaluation' can mean quality measurement, service quality evaluation, evaluation of a quality system, evaluation of a quality programme and research quality evaluation.
- Both measurement and evaluation involve value judgements about which aspects of quality to measure, but evaluation also involves comparisons over time or between services to judge the value of the measured level of quality performance achieved by a service.
- To design a quality evaluation, evaluators can draw on resources which include definitions and specifications of quality, audit systems and a variety of evaluation methods and published studies which provide examples. However, evaluators need to resist proposing an approach before clarifying the needs of the evaluation user and how they would use the findings.
- Qualefficiency is using the fewest resources to achieve a consistent standard of care, which meets a defined number of patients' essential health needs and wants. By relating quality to the resources available to a service, qualefficiency evaluations provide a more integrated performance measure and allow fairer comparisons. They enable providers to work on reducing waste and errors as well as improving clinical quality and patient satisfaction.

Chapter 14

Evaluation paradigms and perspectives

How can you properly evaluate a service without objectively measuring outcome and controlling for the other explanations for the outcome apart from the service?

How can you properly evaluate a health programme or reform without investigating patients' and providers' subjective experiences?

Introduction

Evaluation aims to produce knowledge about a programme, change or action. All evaluations use systematic data-gathering methods and designs to gather data which can be used to judge the value of the intervention. Beyond this the two main evaluation paradigms – the positivist and the phenomenological – do not have much in common. They hold different assumptions about what is valid evidence and use different methods to gather data.

What does this mean for how we judge the validity of the findings of an evaluation study? Are reports which only give people's subjective views about an intervention not to be trusted? This chapter proposes two tests of validity of the evidence produced by an evaluation: are the findings valid for the user's decisions, and are the findings valid according to the tests of method which are used within a particular scientific paradigm? People's subjective views may or may not be valid evidence, depending on the user's informational needs and on whether accepted methods were used properly.

The book did not discuss these different paradigms earlier because it aimed to give practical and simple guidance. Many of the evaluation designs are used by both approaches, although the randomised controlled trial is the preferred design of the positivist paradigm. The chapter about data-gathering touched on the subject and treated the different methods equally. This chapter now describes these two paradigms so as to give the reader a broader view of evaluation and to promote understanding of why some users' questions are better answered by a positivist and some by a phenomenological evaluation.

The chapter describes the ideas of the positivist and phenomenological paradigms about how to gain knowledge. It illustrates what these ideas mean for practical evaluation in terms of four approaches: the objective, subjective, prospective and retrospective approaches. It then describes the five main evaluation perspectives: the experimental, the economic, the social research, the action evaluation and the managerial approaches.

Positivist and phenomenological paradigms

It is the sort of thing I would not believe, even if it were true.

What counts as evidence of effectiveness? How can we be certain that an intervention really makes a difference? Our answers to these questions depend on our ideas about scientific method and our assumptions about how valid knowledge about interventions and effects is to be gained. We need to understand our own and others' assumptions to understand why some 'qualitative evaluations' are not considered to be research or of value for making decisions by some, and to understand the evidence-based healthcare debate about what is evidence.

This debate has practical consequences. If we conclude that valid evidence can only be produced by using objective measures and controlled trials, then this means that we will not accept many findings from evaluations of health programmes and reforms using other methods. It is not just a question of which methods produce more certain knowledge. The dominant scientific paradigm in healthcare effectively excludes many evaluations of community nursing programmes, alternative medicine and health policies. These are difficult to evaluate using objective measures and controlled trials and, where this is possible, these methods will not capture features of outcome which may be important. It also excludes much evidence from evaluations of health reforms. This is convenient for politicians who do not want debate to be confused by evidence of any type. Who gains from the prevailing view about what is valid evidence? Is it the community nursing service and primary care or specialist medicine, drug manufacturers and many politicians?

If we are evaluating a treatment or drug, the usual approach is to decide which outcomes to measure and study human beings as physical objects. We try to exclude all subjective factors, by blinding and through using a placebo, and we study whether the intervention has an effect on an objective measure such as blood pressure or infection rate. Some medical evaluations do consider the patients' perceptions of benefit, but these are measured as objectively as possible without allowing patients to explore and explain their perceptions and their views are usually viewed as independent of the clinical effects.

When we consider health programmes, policies, reforms or education programmes, we can apply the same approach. If we think of a person as a physical object we concentrate on biochemical, physiological and physical processes which operate according to general laws and can be understood in terms of causation. There are those who think that this way of knowing should be applied to evaluating health programmes, policies and reforms. For example, we can concentrate on objectively measurable outcomes (e.g. costs) and treat the intervention and the targets as if they were physical objects which operate according to causal mechanisms which act independently of human consciousness. This 'natural science' approach has a long history in health research and has been characterised as 'positivist'. It involves assumptions about the nature of 'facts' and about how empirical and explanatory knowledge of the 'real world' can be produced.

Empiricism holds that 'facts speak for themselves' and that the real world can be comprehended directly. Positivism is a development of empiricism and holds that we need pre-observational concepts to help us then gather data directly from the real world (Popper, 1959). Our aim is to gather data to refute hypotheses derived from theory and in this way to build up knowledge of increasing certainty. Objectivity lies in the researcher's detachment from the subject of study, their value neutrality and the accuracy of their data collection. This perspective is most often applied to investigating diseases and influences on health at the individual and population level.

Yet we can also think of a person as a human subject, in the sense of being able to give meaning and value to their experiences and to events in the world. The 'subjectivist' or phenomenological approach holds that, in many areas of existence, individuals can choose to act in different ways and are not governed by causal influences. This approach to health research argues that, to explain both individual acts and many social phenomena, we have to understand how people interpret events. That we should not just view people and social processes as if they were physical objects, but view the intervention as a social process and the 'targets' as individual and collective human subjects actively interpreting and responding to the intervention.

The phenomenological paradigm views valid data about human beings and social groups as data about subjective meanings. Within this paradigm, explanations about how an intervention works must make reference to the perceptions and meanings which people construct. In evaluations we should investigate how people perceive the intervention and the effects, and their perceptions have an objective reality and force regardless of whether these perceptions are 'true'. We also need to understand subjective meanings and actions in terms of a particular environment and culture which makes them intelligible. For example, a hospital merger may 'fail' according to objective measures such as lower costs and higher quality, but to understand how the intervention (the merger) operates we need to understand the cultures of the hospitals and the subjective meaning which people give to the merger.

> *What people think about a health reform is an outcome and an objective reality. People's perceptions are also 'causal mechanisms' influencing the reform outcomes. For many purposes, an evaluation must consider people's perceptions if it is to adequately document outcomes and explain how these outcomes came about.*

Evaluators holding these assumptions would, for example, want to investigate the perceptions which health providers and managers held about the external environment to their programme and how this affected their decisions and how the programme operated. They would collect data about the intervention and its effects and construct explanations in a different way from evaluators working within the positivist paradigm.

There is debate about which approach is 'best' for studying social phenomena and social entities such as hospitals, health policies and health systems. Should these subjects be studied using natural science methods and should we seek to explain events in terms of laws and causation? Or should they be studied using methods to discover the subjective perceptions and values of individuals and groups and explain events in terms of how people give meaning to the events?

The approach taken in this book is not to argue for or against a particular paradigm but to highlight the issues. Each approach can bring insights: for example, a disease process in an individual can be understood in terms of the subjective meanings given to the disease by the person, which in turn is influenced by their culture. These meanings may even affect the course of the disease, but the disease also progresses on a predictable course which can be illuminated by taking a natural science perspective. The same applies to a health programme or implementing a policy or a reform.

Generally this book takes a 'dualist' or mixed approach: that people and social groups are influenced by factors about which they may not be aware and which may have a causal effect on them which show law-like regularities. But individuals and social groups are also able to understand some of these influences and to choose not to be determined by some or to accommodate to others and give meaning to these influences.

Types of evaluation

The following shows how the different assumptions described above translate into different types of evaluation. The results of an intervention can be studied both by asking what people think and without asking their views. Which approach you use depends on the user's questions and informational needs and your disciplinary background and methodological skills. To evaluate a health programme or a change, should we gather objective measures only or also people's subjective perceptions? Should we do a prospective experimental evaluation or a retrospective quasi-experimental evaluation or a 'social evaluation'? The following describes the choices facing an evaluator between four types of evaluation.

Choice 1: prospective experimental evaluation 2 (design type 3,4,5)

This type of evaluation aims to test a hypothesis that the intervention does not have an effect or less effect compared to the alternative. Examples are an evaluation of two back pain progammes or of a new financing system for hospitals compared to the old. The prospective experimental evaluation looks forwards and plans data gathering and controls before the intervention is carried out.

$$\text{Target} \rightarrow \text{M1} \rightarrow \text{Intervention} \rightarrow \text{M2} \rightarrow$$

Before (objective measures)   After (objective measures)

The questions addressed by this type of evaluation are as follows.

- Is the 'before' measure of the target variable different from the 'after' measure (e.g. cost per patient is $250 before and $220 after)?

- Why? What are the other explanations for this difference, apart from the intervention? (Was it the new testing equipment (the intervention) or the change in type of nurses or other changes which explain the lower average cost?)

Choice 2: prospective quanti-qualitative

This is the same as the above but in addition to collecting objective measures, the evaluator plans and then collects the subjective perceptions of selected informants, both before and after. Examples might be subjective perceptions of pain in a treatment evaluation or the perceptions of one group of patients about the quality of a service before a reform compared to the perceptions of a comparable group after the reform.

Choice 3: retrospective subjective

In this type of evaluation the evaluator looks back in time at an intervention which has been completed or is still in progress. The evaluator asks different informants to give their opinions about the results of the intervention. The evaluation users are presented with the assessments made by different informants and the evaluator's summary of the pattern of the evidence.

This approach can be used to give users feedback about a health programme or about a change which is being implemented. For example, a reform may have been started in 1999 and is expected to finish or continue into 2002 but the users want an evaluation to report by 2001. The evaluator would discuss with the users which information they want and select informants from a cross-section of people. They would ask informants to describe what they understood the reform objectives to be, what had been done, what the results were and to predict other results. There would be no controls, but the evaluator would collect data to describe the environment and other possible 'causes' of any results which are described.

Choice 4: retrospective quali-quantitative

This approach is the same as the above but also includes objective data about the target population or organisation before the intervention and objective data about the intervention. The sources of these data are administrative or clinical records and other types of documentation. The evaluator would search for 'good informants' who could describe the intervention and give a view of the results of the intervention, but who could also suggest any 'evidence' which may exist to support their view or which may conflict with it. The evaluator would also ask whether any other events could have produced the results which the informants attribute to the intervention.

Evaluation approaches

Evaluators bring to their task assumptions about what is valid knowledge, their skills in using certain methods to gather data and a view about their role and what an evaluation should do. All this can be summarised as 'an approach' to evaluation and there are a number of different approaches. An 'evaluation approach' is the way an evaluator approaches making an evaluation: it is a combination of the perspective they take – what they see and do not see – and the purpose of the evaluation – who and what it is for (e.g. to produce scientific knowledge or to inform practical decisions). Those noted below are the experimental, the economic, the social research, the action evaluation and the managerial approaches to evaluation.

An evaluation perspective both 'sees' and 'focuses' on certain aspects of an intervention or policy and on its consequences. For example, an economic perspective focuses on how many resources are used by an intervention and the benefits produced by it. A perspective carries assumptions about whether what we can see really exists: it involves assumptions about what is valid knowledge about the aspects of the intervention which are selected and about how to create this knowledge (methodology). These assumptions frame how the evaluator conceptualises the intervention and shapes the evaluation design and the data-gathering and analysis methods.

Box 14.1: Five evaluation approaches

- *Experimental*: tests predictions, controls confounders, a preference for objective measures of outcome
- *Economic*: quantifies the resources consumed by the intervention and the benefits of the consequences
- *Social research evaluation*: describes the intervention and gathers data from many sources about inputs, process and sometimes also outcomes

- *Action evaluation*: the evaluator collaborates with evaluation users and service providers to collect data to answer their questions, sometimes changing the intervention whilst the evaluation is being done
- *Managerial*: inspection or assessing performance for accountability purposes or to improve the functioning of a programme or reform

Experimental

Experimental evaluations aim to discover whether an intervention has effects and sometimes also the causes. There is the prospective and the retrospective experimental approach. Most evaluations of this type use objective measures of the before-and-after state of the target. The evaluation is designed to test hypotheses and follows the model of a scientific experiment. The intervention is carefully defined and held stable. Attempts are made to control for influences other than the intervention which might affect the measured before-and-after variables. The ideal is a prospective experiment because this helps the evaluator to plan and do everything they can to control for influences other than the intervention; for example, using a placebo for the control group which mimics the intervention in everything apart from the active ingredient.

The blinded randomised controlled trial is the ideal design because it helps to exclude influences which the evaluator may not know about or cannot predict. It does this by randomly allocating patients or target subjects and by ensuring that patients, providers and researchers do not know which subjects are in the control and which are in the placebo group. Retrospective experimental evaluations are not real experiments but use the same principles. This approach, used in epidemiological evaluations, treats the intervention to which the targets are exposed as an experiment and looks retrospectively at data which may be available before and after the 'exposure intervention'.

At the other extreme there are experimental evaluation designs used in quality improvement projects. A project team may analyse a quality problem, such as operation cancellations, and decide certain changes to improve quality, for example better operation scheduling. The team would carry out the changes as an experiment and collect data to find out if the change had an effect (Øvretveit, 2000a).

A variety of designs are used but all involve the idea of an experiment, a defined hypothesis which is tested, maximising control of the intervention and of other possible influences, and one or a few objective measures. Evaluations of this type are usually carried out within a positivist paradigm. However, not all just collect data from objective measures: more are now collecting data about people's subjective perceptions. Although most are carried out by external and detached evaluator-researchers, some experimental evaluations are carried out by people internal to the organisation or by quality project teams.

Economic

Economic evaluations aim to discover how many resources are consumed by using an intervention and usually also to quantify the consequences of an intervention, sometimes in money terms. Economic evaluations share many of the assumptions of the experimental paradigm about objective measurement and controls and are often built on experimental evaluations. For example, a common type of economic evaluation would try to quantify the resources used in a health programme and express these in money terms. It would try to measure the consequences of the programme and express these in terms of the resources saved and consumed. There are different ways to quantify consequences, such as increase in length of life, decrease in morbidity and quality of life.

For option appraisal the economic approach is to estimate:

- the cost of not intervening
- the 'spend cost' of making the intervention
- the likely savings at one year and five years.

The intervention would be considered 'low price' if the benefits exceeded the costs or effort (Øvretveit, 2000b). The economic approach to evaluation assumes that the resources used could always be put to other uses and tries to compare the costs and consequences of the intervention to those of other ways of using the resources (Drummond *et al.*, 1987).

Social research evaluations

This approach is the one most commonly used to evaluate health policies and reforms and many programmes. It draws on a social research tradition, uses descriptive and non-experimental naturalistic or quasi-experimental designs and a variety of data-gathering methods and the evaluators keep a 'respectful distance' from the intervention. Some evaluations within this approach attempt to get evidence about outcome, but do so without the rigorous controls or techniques to reduce bias of the full experimental evaluation or of the single-case experimental design. Social research evaluations often use case study methods (Yin, 1989) and are carried out using social policy research methods.

There is a fine dividing line between some social research and quasi-experimental evaluations. There is a spectrum of social research evaluations ranging from those close to the experimental paradigm to, at the other extreme, those working with phenomenological and naturalistic methods. The latter aim to give service providers or policy makers feedback which they can use to change and improve a service or intervention.

Action evaluation

Another approach draws on an action research tradition (Hart and Bond, 1996; Lewin, 1947a, b) with the evaluator working closely with users, providers and patients. Action evaluations use systematic methods and theories within an evaluation framework to enable service providers or other evaluation users to develop and improve their programmes, policies or organisational interventions. For example, in one type of action evaluation, the evaluators might interview ten patients two weeks before they receive a service and at two weeks after, to find out what they expected and how they were involved in treatment decisions. The findings would be reported back to the service providers by the evaluator who would work with them to decide ways to improve patient involvement.

Action evaluations have an immediate practical focus and involve the evaluator working in an independent role with evaluation users and providers to enable users to judge the value of the intervention or providers to assess and improve what they are doing. Action evaluations may also be carried out by providers themselves for self-improvement or in a peer review process.

Action evaluations often aim to help providers to change their progamme or reform whilst the evaluation is being made (Øvretveit, 1987). These type of evaluations are at the other end of a spectrum of 'control' from where experimental RCT evaluations would be placed. They do not always evaluate a service against objectives or criteria, but some action evaluations may help the service or others develop such objectives or criteria. It is the collaborative, practical, direct and immediate working with evaluation users and service providers, but with the evaluator in an independent role, which distinguishes the action evaluation from other types (Øvretveit, 1998a).

Both social research and action evaluations are useful for evaluating the many changes and programmes where:

- the objectives and boundaries of the change or programme are unclear
- there is complex and continual change in the change or programme intervention
- there is uncertainty about the effects of the change or intervention and about what might cause the effects
- users want more knowledge quickly.

But these approaches may be less useful for evaluating a health programme which is established and stable. They are not suitable when users want limited but certain information about the effects, in order to compare the value of the programme with a comparison.

Managerial evaluations

Managerial evaluations are made for managers and supervisory boards to monitor or improve the performance of services or policies or to check that agreed changes or projects were implemented as intended. Their purpose is to ensure accountability, value for money and performance improvement. For example, one type of managerial evaluation might involve evaluators sending people a short questionnaire to find out if they are aware of a health programme. Another may be an audit inspection to check if a hospital has a system for ensuring quality and gives a report on areas for improvement. Many managerial evaluations in health compare actual activities against procedures and standards which are thought to ensure safety, efficiency, effectiveness and equity. They are usually done by people working for health service organisations, although external evaluators may be used to help create systems for audit or for performance management evaluations.

Conclusion

There are a few points to be made in conclusion. First, there are different and strongly held views within the multidiscipline of evaluation about how to evaluate health interventions. Second, this book proposed that there is a place for all perspectives and approaches. Which you use depends on your training, the purpose and questions to be answered and on what would be most credible to the users of the evaluation. The third point is to note that this 'live and let live' approach is not shared by many evaluators and this is especially apparent in debates about interventions which lie on the boundaries between a treatment and a service, as for example in some combined cancer treatments. This book proposed a user-focused approach as the one most likely to produce findings that can be acted on. Many of the chapters aimed to show how to follow a user-focused approach in making an evaluation. Whether you evaluate your own service or practice or someone else's health programme or change, I know that you will find these ideas useful. The work and the fun is in applying the ideas. Use your skills to make a difference which benefits others.

Summary

- Evaluations performed within either the positivist or phenomenological paradigm can produce valid or invalid findings. Validity in evaluation depends on whether the evaluation uses the methods of the paradigm correctly and on whether the findings are relevant to the user's informational needs.
- The assumptions of the positivist paradigm are that valid knowledge is produced by testing predictions about objectively measurable phenomena. In evaluation this means viewing the intervention as an experiment and gathering data using objective measures.
- The assumptions of the phenomenological paradigm are that valid knowledge about human beings and social processes is produced by finding out how people perceive and make sense of phenomena. In evaluation this means selecting informants and trying to fully understand what they think and feel about an intervention and its effects.
- Both produce valid knowledge about an intervention and its effects if the methods which are accepted within the paradigm are used correctly and if the knowledge is relevant to the users' needs.
- Four different approaches illustrate these paradigms applied within evaluation:
  1 prospective experimental evaluations which gather objective measures before and after
  2 prospective evaluations which also gather data about the target's subjective experiences
  3 retrospective subjective evaluations which gather the perceptions of different informants about the intervention and its effects
  4 retrospective quali-quantitative evaluations which gather both subjective and objective data.

- There are five evaluation approaches which have evolved in response to users' needs and through evaluators drawing on their scientific disciplines to meet these needs. These are the experimental, the economic, the social research, the action evaluation and the managerial approaches to making an evaluation.

References

Adams G and Shvaneveldt J (1991) *Understanding Research Methods.* Longman, New York.

Alban A and Christiansen T (eds) (1995) *The Nordic Lights: new initiatives in health care systems.* Odense University Press, Odense.

Aletras V, Jones A and Sheldon T (1997) Economies of scale and scope. In: B Ferguson, T Sheldon and J Posnet (eds) *Concentration and Choice in Healthcare.* Financial Times Healthcare, London.

Anell A and Svarvar P (1993) Reformed county council model. IHE Working Paper, Lund.

Babakus E and Mangold WG (1992) Adapting the SERVQUAL scale to hospital services: an empirical investigation. *Health Services Res.* **26**(6): 767–86.

Bergman S (1998) Swedish models of healthcare reform: a reveiw and assessment. *Int J Health Planning Management.* **13**: 91–106.

Bero L, Grilli R, Grimshaw J *et al.* (1998) Closing the gap between research and practice: an overview of systematic reviews of interventions to promote the implementation of research findings. *BMJ.* **317**: 465–8.

Berwick D, Godfrey A and Roessner J (1990) *Curing Healthcare: new strategies for quality improvement.* Jossey-Bass, San Francisco.

Black N (1992) Research, audit and education. *BMJ.* **304**: 698–700.

Blumenthal D and Scheck A (eds) (1995) *Improving Clinical Practice: total quality management and the physician.* Jossey-Bass, San Francisco.

Bowling A (1992) *Measuring Health: a review of quality of life measures.* Open University Press, Milton Keynes.

Bowling A (1995) *Measuring Disease: a review of disease-specific quality of life measurement scales.* Open University Press, Milton Keynes.

Breakwell G and Millward L (1995) *Basic Evaluation Methods.* British Psychological Society Books, Leicester.

Britten N (1995) Qualitative interviews in medical research. *BMJ.* **311**: 251–3.

Brogren P and Brommels M (1990) Central and local control in Nordic health care. *Int J Health Planning Management.* **5**: 27–39.

Brooks T (1992) Success through organisational audit. *Health Services Management.* **Nov/Dec**: 13–5.

Crombie I (1996) *The Pocket Guide to Critical Appraisal.* BMJ Books, London.

Daly J, McDonald I and Willis E (eds) (1992) *Researching Health Care: designs, dilemmas, disciplines*. Routledge, London.

Denzin N and Lincoln Y (eds) (1994) *Handbook of Qualitative Research*. Sage, London.

DHHSPHS (1995) *Performance Improvement 1995: evaluation activities of the public health services*. US Department of Health and Human Services, Washington DC.

Donabedian A (1980) *Exploration in Quality Assessment and Monitoring Volume I: definition of quality and approaches to its assessment*. Health Administration Press, University of Michigan, Ann Arbor.

Drummond M, Stoddard G and Torrence G (1987) *Methods for the Economic Evaluation of Health Care Programmes*. Oxford Medical Publications, Oxford.

Edgren L (1995) *Evaluation of the SPRI Version of Organisational Audit at Lund University Hospital*. Nordic School of Public Health, Goteborg (summary in English).

Edwards A and Talbot R (1994) *The Hard-Pressed Researcher*. Longman, London.

EGGE (1999) Guidelines for evaluating papers on educational interventions. *BMJ*. **318**: 1265–6.

Ekberg K, Bjorkqvist IK, Malm B *et al.* (1994) Controlled two year follow-up of rehabilitation for disorders in the neck and shoulders. *Occup Environ Med.* **51**: 833–8.

Fink A (1993) *Evaluation Fundamentals*. Sage, London.

Fitzpatrick R and Boulton M (1994) Qualitative methods for assessing health care. *Quality in Health Care*. **3**: 107–13.

Frankfort-Nachmias C and Nachmias D (1992) *Research Methods in Social Sciences (4e)*. Edward Arnold, London.

Gardner M and Altman D (1989) *Statistics with Confidence*. BMJ Books, London.

Ghauri P, Grønhaug K and Kristianslund I (1995) *Research Methods in Business Studies*. Prentice-Hall, London.

Glaser BG and Strauss AL (1968) *The Discovery of Grounded Theory: strategies for qualitative research*. Weidenfeld and Nicolson, London.

Golden B (1992) The past is the past – or is it? The use of retrospective accounts as indicators of past strategy. *Acad Management J*. **35**(4): 848–60.

Gray M (1997) *Evidence-Based Healthcare*. Churchill Livingstone, London.

Greene J (1994) Qualitative program evaluation. In: N Denzin and Y Lincoln (eds) *Handbook of Qualitative Research*. Sage, London.

Greenhalgh J, Long A, Brettle A and Grant M (1996) The value of an outcomes information resource. *J Management Med*. **10**(5): 55–65.

Greenhalgh T (1997) Assessing the methodological quality of published papers. *BMJ*. **315**: 305–8.

Hakkinen U (1997) The changing roles of municipalities in Finnish health care. *Eurohealth*. **4**(1): 18–21.

Hart E and Bond M (1996) *Action Research for Health and Social Care*. Open University Press, Milton Keynes.

Hawe P, Degeling D and Hull J (1990) *Evaluating Health Promotion*. Maclennan and Petty, London.

Haynes B and Haines A (1998) Barriers and bridges to evidence based clinical practice. *BMJ*. **317**: 273.

HERG (1994) *Assessing Payback from Department of Health Research and Development*. Health Economics Research Group, Brunel University, Uxbridge.

Heron J (1986) Critique of conventional research methodology. *Complementary Med Res*. **1**(1): 14–22.

House E (1980) *Evaluating with Validity*. Sage, Beverly Hills.

JCSEE (1994) *The Programme Evaluation Standards: how to assess evaluations of educational programs (2e)*. Sage, Thousand Oaks.

Jick T (1983) Mixing qualitative and quantitative methods: triangulation in action. In: J Van Maanen (ed) *Qualitative Methodology*. Sage, Beverly Hills.

Joss R and Kogan M (1995) *Advancing Quality*. Open University Press, Milton Keynes.

Joss R, Kogan M and Henkel M (1994) *Final Report to the Department of Health on Total Quality Management Experiments in the National Health Service*. Centre for Evaluation of Public Policy and Practice, Brunel University.

JRF (2001) *Communication and Consultation*. Joseph Rowntree Foundation, York.

Kitson A, Harvey G, Hyndman S *et al.* (1994) *The Impact of a Nursing Quality Assurance Approach, The Dynamic Standard Setting System (DySSSy), on Nursing Practice and Patient Outcomes. The ODySSSy Project*. National Institute for Nursing, Oxford.

Kitzinger J (1995) Introducing focus groups. *BMJ*. **311**: 299–302.

Kreuger R (1988) *Focus Groups: a practical guide for applied research*. Sage, London.

Kvale S (1994) Ten standard objections to qualitative research interviews. *J Phenomenological Psychol*. 1–28.

Lawrence M and Packwood T (1996) Adapting total quality management for general practice: evaluation of a programme. *Quality in Health Care*. **5**: 151–8.

Lewin K (1947a) Group decision and social change. In: T Newcomb and E Hartley (eds) *Readings in Social Psychology*. Holt, Rinehart and Winston, New York.

Lewin K (1947b) Frontiers in group dynamics: 1) concept, methods and reality in social sciences: social equilibria and social change, 2) channels of group life, social planning and action research. *Human Relations*. **1**(1, 2): 5–41, 143–53.

Lincoln Y and Guba E (1985) *Naturalistic Inquiry*. Sage, Newbury Park.

Maxwell R (1984) Quality assessment in health. *BMJ*. **288**: 1470–2.

McConway K (ed) (1994) *Studying Health and Disease*. Open University Press, Milton Keynes.

McKinlay J (1992) Advantages and limitations of the survey approach – understanding older people. In Daly J, McDonald I and Willis E (eds) *Researching Health Care*. Routledge, London.

Menckel E and Westerholm P (eds) (1999) *Evaluation and Development of Occupational Health Practice: a handbook for occupational health service professionals*. Arbetslivsinstitutet, Solna, Sweden.

Miles M and Huberman A (1994) *Qualitative Data Analysis: a source book of new methods (2e)*. Sage, Beverly Hills.

Morgan D (ed) (1993) *Successful Focus Groups*. Sage, London.

Nathanson C (1978) Sex roles as a variable in the interpretation of morbidity data: a methodological critique. *Int J Epidemiol*. **7**(3): 253–62.

NCEPOD (1987, 1989) *Report of a National Confidential Enquiry into Perioperative Deaths*. King's Fund, London.

NCEPOD (1993) *Report of the National Confidential Enquiry into Perioperative Deaths, 1991/92*. King's Fund, London.

Nelson E and Batalden P (1993) Patient-based quality measurement systems. *Quality Management in Health Care*. **2**(1): 18–30.

Nelson E, Batalden P, Plume S and Mohr J (1996) Improving health care part 2: a clinical improvement worksheet and users' manual. *J Quality Improvement*. **22**(8): 531–48.

Newman D and Brown R (1998) *Applied Ethics for Program Evaluation*. Sage, London.

Øvretveit J (1986) *Improving Social Work Records and Practice*. BASW Publications, Birmingham.

Øvretveit J (1987) Volunteers in drugs agencies: an evaluation of supervision arrangements. BIOSS Working Paper, Brunel University, Uxbridge.

Øvretveit J (1991a) *Primary Care Quality Through Teamwork*. Research Report, BIOSS, Brunel University, Uxbridge.

Øvretveit J (1991b) Quality costs – or does it? *Health Service Management*. **August**: 184–5.

Øvretveit J (1992a) *Health Service Quality*. Blackwell Science, Oxford.

Øvretveit J (1992b) Towards market-focused measures of customer/purchaser perceptions. *Quality Forum*. **19**(3): 21–4.

Øvretveit J (1993) *Measuring Service Quality*. Technical Communications Publications, Aylesbury.

Øvretveit J (1994a) A comparison of approaches to quality in the UK, USA and

Sweden, and of the use of organisational audit frameworks. *Eur J Public Health.* **4**(1): 46–54.

Øvretveit J (1994b) *Purchasing for Health.* Open University Press, Milton Keynes.

Øvretveit J (1997) Assessing evaluations of hospital quality programmes. *Evaluation.* **3**(4): 451–68.

Øvretveit J (1998a) *Evaluating Health Interventions.* Open University Press, Milton Keynes.

Øvretveit J (1998b) *Comparative and Cross Cultural Health Research.* Radcliffe Medical Press, Oxford.

Øvretveit J (1999) *Integrated Quality Development for Public Healthcare.* Norwegian Medical Association, Oslo, Norway.

Øvretveit J (2000a) The team quality improvement sequence. *Quality in Health Care.* **8**: 1–7.

Øvretveit J (2000b) The economics of quality – a practical approach. *Int J Health Care Quality Assurance.* **13**(5): 200–7.

Øvretveit J and Aslaksen A (1999) *The Quality Journeys of Six Norwegian Hospitals.* Norwegian Medical Association, Oslo, Norway.

Patton M (1980) *Qualitative Evaluation Methods.* Sage, London.

Patton M (1987) *How to Use Qualitative Methods in Evaluation.* Sage, London.

Phillips C, Palfry C and Thomas, P (1994) *Evaluating Health and Social Care.* Macmillan, London.

Pope C and Mays N (1995a) Observational methods in health care settings. *BMJ.* **311**: 182–4.

Pope C and Mays N (1995b) Reaching the parts other methods cannot reach: an introduction to qualitative methods in health and health services research. *BBMJ.* **311**: 42–5.

Popper K (1959) *The Logic of Scientific Discovery.* Hutchinson, London.

Posnett J (1999) Is bigger better? Concentration in the provision of secondary care. *BMJ.* **319**: 1063–5.

Powell J, Lovelock R, Bray J and Philp I (1994) Involving consumers in assessing service quality using a qualitative approach. *Quality in Health Care.* **3**: 199–202.

Robinson R and Le Grand J (1994) *Evaluating the NHS Reforms.* King's Fund Institute, London.

Rossi P and Freeman H (1993) *Evaluation – a systematic approach.* Sage, London.

Rossi P and Wright S (1977) Evaluation research: an assessment of theory, practice and politics. *Evaluation Quarterly.* **1**: 5–52.

Sackett D, Rosenberg W, Gray J, Haynes R and Scott-Richardson W (1996) Evidence-based medicine: what it is and what it isn't. *BMJ.* **312**: 71–2.

Saltman R and Figueras J (1997) *European Healthcare Reform*. WHO, Copenhagen.

Saltman R, Figueras J and Sakellarides C (eds) (1998) *Critical Challenges for Healthcare Reform in Europe*. Open University Press, Milton Keynes.

Sapsford R and Abbott P (1992) *Research Methods for Nurses and the Caring Professions*. Open University Press, Milton Keynes.

Scott D and Weston R (1998) *Evaluating Health Promotion*. Stanley Thornes, Cheltenham.

Scriven M (1991) *Evaluation Thesaurus*. Sage, London.

Statens Helsitilsyn (1995) *Nasjonal strategi for kvalitetsutvikling i heslsetjenesten*. Statens helsetilsyn, Oslo (No. 1K 2482). (English translation available)

Smith M, Glass G and Miller T (1980) *The Benefits of Psychotherapy*. Johns Hopkins University Press, Baltimore.

St Leger A, Schienden H and Walsworth-Bell J (1992) *Evaluating Health Service Effectiveness*. Open University Press, Milton Keynes.

Stern E (1990) *Evaluating Innovatory Programmes*. The Tavistock Institute, London.

Stern E (1993) The challenge of 'real-time' evaluation. In: *The Tavistock Institute Review 1992–93*. The Tavistock Institute, London.

Strauss A and Corbin J (1990) *Basics of Qualitative Research*. Sage, London.

Van De Vijver F and Leung K (1997) *Methods and Data Analysis for Cross-Cultural Research*. Sage, London.

Weiss C (ed) (1977) *Using Social Research in Public Policy Making*. Lexington Books, Mass.

Weiss C (1978) Improving the linkage between social research and public policy. In: L Lynn (ed) *Knowledge and Policy: the uncertain connection*. National Academy of Sciences, Washington DC.

WHO (1981) *Health Programme Evaluation*. World Health Organisation, Geneva.

WHO (1994) *Implementation of the Global Strategy for Health for All by the Year 2000 – Second Evaluation. Eighth Report of the World Health Situation*. World Health Organisation, Geneva. (Note: volume 5 is the European Region Report. First evaluation was in 1988.)

WHO (1996) *Health Care Reforms in Europe*. World Health Organisation, Copenhagen.

Wiltkin D, Hallan L and Dogget M (1992) *Measures of Need and Outcome for Primary Health Care*. Oxford Medical Publications, Oxford.

Yin R (1981) The case study crisis: some answers. *Admin Sci Quart.* **26**(1): 58–65.

Yin R (1989) *Case Study Research: design and methods*. Sage, Beverly Hills.

Definitions

Action evaluation: is carried out for one user group using their value criteria and provides them with data to make more informed decisions. The evaluator works with the evaluation user to clarify the criteria to be used to judge the value of an intervention, as well as to clarify the decisions which the user has to make which can be informed by the evaluation. It is collaborative, usually gathers people's subjective perceptions, is carried out in a short time and provides actionable data for the evaluation users.

Action research: a systematic investigation which aims to contribute to knowledge as well as solve a practical problem.

Audit: an investigation into whether an activity meets explicit standards as defined by an auditing document. The auditing process can be carried out by external auditors or internally for self-review and can use external ready-made audit standards or internally developed standards. Medical and clinical audit is using pre-existing standards or setting standards comparing practice with standards and changing practice if necessary and is usually carried out internally for self-review and improvement. Peer audit can use already existing standards or practitioners can develop their own, but usually practitioners adapt existing standards to their own situation.

'Blinding': single-blinded trail: the people in the control and experimental groups (subjects) do not know which group they are in.

'Blinding': double-blinded trail: neither the subjects nor the service providers know which group is the experimental and which is the control.

'Box': the boundary around the intervention, which defines what is evaluated and separates it from the environment. Includes inside the box a specification of the components of the intervention.

Case control study: a retrospective observational study of people or organisations with a particular characteristic ('cases') compared to those which do not have this characteristic (controls), to find out possible causes or influences which could explain the characteristic.

Case study: 'attempts to examine a contemporary phenomenon in its real-life context, especially when the boundaries between context and phenomenon are not clearly evident' (Yin, 1981).

Cohort: a group of people, usually sharing one or more characteristics, who are followed over time to find out what happens to them.

Confounding factors or variables: something other than the intervention which could influence the measured outcome.

Continuous quality improvement: an approach for ensuring that staff continually improve work processes by using proven quality methods to discover and resolve the causes of quality problems in a systematic way.

Control group or control site: a group of people or an organisation which does not get the intervention. The evaluation compares them to the experimental group or site, which gets the intervention. People are randomly allocated to either group or, if this is not possible, the control group or site is 'matched' with the experimental group.

Cost-benefit: valuing the consequences of a programme in money terms, so as to compare the assessed value with the actual costs. A range of benefits are valued in money terms.

Cost description: measurement of the costs of one thing, or of more than one, in a way which allows an explicit or implicit comparison of costs. (A 'partial' economic evaluation looks at only one intervention and does not make an explicit comparison.)

Cost-effectiveness: the effectiveness or consequences, as shown by one measure (e.g. lives saved, cases of diseases avoided or years of healthy life) compared with the cost. No attempt is made to value the consequences – it is assumed that the output is of value. Used to compare the different costs of using different ways to achieve the same end result.

Cost minimisation: assumes that the differences in outcome produced by the alternatives are not significant and calculates the cost of each alternative with the purpose of discovering which is the lowest cost.

Cost-utility: considers the utility of the end result to the patient for the cost. Often uses the QALY measure. Measures consequences in time units adjusted by health utility weights (i.e. states of health associated with outcome are valued relative to each other). More complex than cost-effectiveness.

Criterion: a comparison against which we judge the intervention – effectiveness is an example of such a criterion.

Evaluation: judging the value of something by gathering information about it in a systematic way and by making a comparison, for the purpose of making a better informed decision. (Other definitions are given at the end of this appendix.)

Evaluated: the action or intervention which is evaluated – the subject of the evaluation.

Evaluation-informed management (EIM): making more informed management decisions by using research evidence and evidence from inside the organisation and making more effective actions and projects by using evaluation concepts to plan management interventions.

Evaluator: the person doing the evaluation.

Evidence-based medicine: 'the conscientious, explicit, and judicious use of current best evidence in making decisions about the care of individual patients. The practice of EBM means integrating individual clinical expertise with best available external clinical evidence from systematic research' (Sackett *et al.*, 1996).

External evaluators: research or consultancy units not directly managed by and independent from the sponsor and user of the evaluation.

Internal evaluators: evaluation and development units which are internal to the organisation, who evaluate treatments, services or policies carried out by the organisation or one of its divisions.

Intervention: an action on or attempt to change a person, population or organisation, which is the subject of an evaluation (e.g. a health service, programme, policy or reform).

ISO 9000: a description of how an organisation should write down in a quality manual ('documentation') its arrangements for allocating responsibility for quality, how it should define objectives, policies and procedures and how the organisation then ensures that these arrangements are followed (control) and poor quality is recorded. ISO 9000 is a 'standard' for a 'quality system'.

Matching: ensuring that people (or organisations) in the experimental and control groups (or sites) are the same, in all the characteristics which could affect the outcome of the intervention which is given to the experimental group or site.

Monitoring: continuous supervision of an activity to check whether plans and procedures are being followed. (Audit is a subtype of the wider activity of monitoring.)

Operationalise: converting something general (e.g. a criterion) into something specific, usually into something which we can measure (e.g. a measure of amount of sleep such as a diary record).

Organisational audit: an external inspection of aspects of a service, in comparison to established standards, and a review of an organisation's arrangements to control and assure the quality of its products or services. Audits use criteria (or "standards") against which auditors judge elements of a service's planning, organisation, systems and performance.

Outcome: the difference an intervention makes to the person, population or organisation which is the target of the intervention.

Outcome measure: a measure of an important predicted effect of the intervention on the target person or population.

Patient pathway: a description and diagram of the series of steps over time taken by a patient passing to and through different services when seeking help for a health problem (Øvretveit, 1994a). The pathway may be a simple diagram of decisions at different stages (patient flow diagram) or it may be a more detailed checklist and record of tasks to be done at different stages (e.g. critical path, integrated care pathway, anticipated recovery path, care plan, care protocols, care paths).
   Pathways are often defined for patients with a particular type of health condition or diagnosis where their care is predictable and standardisation can reduce unwanted variations in care.

Placebo: something which the subjects of the intervention think is an intervention, but which has no known 'active ingredient' (used to control for effects which may be caused only by subjects thinking that they are receiving an intervention). From the Latin *I will please*.

Police car effect: people who think they are being evaluated follow regulations more closely than when they think that they are not being evaluated.

Procedure/protocol (guideline, routine): a written statement of how to carry out a task. Some procedures give more details about a part of the patient's pathway or part of a process. Some procedures are written by referring to research into effective ways to carry out a treatment (evidence-based procedures/protocols or guidelines).

Process: a sequence of activities which produces a valued change in a person, object or information.

Prospective evaluation: designing an evaluation and then collecting data while the intervention is happening and usually also before and after the intervention.

Public health quality: the ability of a health system to protect and improve the health of a population. It depends on traditional improvements to healthcare services, but also on programmes for those who make little use of these services and whose voice is rarely heard in surveys.

Qualefficiency: using the fewest resources to consistently achieve a standard of care which meets patients' essential health needs and wants.

Quality: meeting the health needs of those most in need at the lowest cost and within regulations (Øvretveit, 1992a).

Quality accreditation: a certification through an external evaluation of whether a practitioner, equipment or a service meets standards which are thought to contribute to quality processes and outcomes.

Quality assurance: a general term for activities and systems for monitoring and improving quality. Quality assurance involves but is more than measuring quality and evaluating quality.

Quality problem: an opportunity to close the gap between how things are and how they could be better.

Quality programme: a set of activities to ensure and develop the quality of a service, which are usually planned and organisation-wide, and include training, providing quality methods expertise, setting up project teams, defining responsibilities for quality and measuring quality.

Quality project: a time-limited task to solve a quality problem or improve quality, undertaken by a specially created team using quality methods in a structured way.

Quality system: a set of requirements which state the actions a healthcare organisation must take to systematically identify and correct quality problems. Many quality systems require the organisation to define responsibilities for quality and the necessary procedures, to ensure these are known to all personnel and that quality performance is documented and corrective action is taken when poor quality occurs. A quality system is a co-ordinated set of procedures, division of responsibilities and processes for setting quality standards and procedures, identifying quality problems and resolving these problems. (BSI 5750 and ISO 9000 are standards for a quality system.)

Randomisation: allocating people in a random way to an experimental or a control group. The purpose is to try to ensure that the people (or organisations) with characteristics which might affect the outcome are allocated evenly to both groups. This is because there are many known and unknown characteristics which may influence outcome. Randomisation allows the evaluators to consider as significant any differences between the two groups which are more than chance differences and avoids the need for matching.

Randomised controlled trial: an experiment where one group gets the intervention and another group does not and people are assigned to both groups in a random way.

Retrospective evaluation: looking into the past for evidence about the intervention ('concurrent' means at the same time).

Research – basic or pure: the use of scientific methods which are appropriate for discovering valid knowledge of a phenomenon for the purpose of contributing to scientific knowledge about the subject.

Review: a single or regular assessment of an activity, which may or may not compare the activity to an explicit plan, criteria or standards. Most audits or monitoring are types of review. Many 'managerial evaluations' are reviews or monitoring.

Self-evaluation: practitioners or teams evaluating their own practice so as to improve it.

Sensitivity: the ability of a test to detect all true positives or of a measure to detect changes in the phenomena being measured.

Specificity: the ability of a test to identify true negatives.

Sponsor: those who initiate or pay for the evaluation.

Stakeholder: a person or group with interests in the outcome of an intervention or an evaluation of it (e.g. patients, citizens, health personnel, managers).

System: a set of elements which interact with each other and which function as a whole to produce an effect. Systems thinking is seeing the connections: understanding that the causes of quality problems are not singular but that different things interact and seeing the solutions as changing interactions and how the whole works, not just changing one thing. Systems management is creating connections and synergy through synchronising and other methods.

System of care quality: the ability of services to co-operate to assess and meet the requirements of the patient, at the lowest costs, without duplication or errors and so that the patient experiences care as one continuous episode.

System of care quality development: combining professional, management and organisational quality methods to develop the 'system of care' experienced by the patient to produce better patient experiences and less patient suffering using fewer resources.

Target: the part or whole of the person or population which the intervention aims to affect.

Total quality management (TQM): a comprehensive strategy of organisational and attitude change for enabling staff to learn and use quality methods in order to reduce costs and meet the requirements of patients and other 'customers'. Quality is 'a method of management'; quality is determined by systems of care and management are responsible for the performance of these systems.

User: those who make use of or act on an evaluation.

Validity (internal): the validity of an evaluation experiment, for example in being able to show whether or not the intervention has an effect or the size of the effect.

Validity (external): the ability of an evaluation experiment to show that the findings would also apply when the intervention was applied in another setting.

Value criterion: what is important to people in how they judge the value of an intervention.

Variable (dependent): the outcome or end result of a treatment service or policy (the main thing the evaluation has to find out about, e.g. lower blood pressure, nurses following a procedure after receiving an educational intervention).

Variable (independent): something which may cause the outcome. Any variable whose effect on another variable is to be assessed.

Evaluation: some different definitions

The process of determining the merit, worth and value of things, and evaluations are the products of that process. (Scriven, 1991)

Program evaluations aim to provide convincing evidence that a program is effective. The standards are the specific criteria by which effectiveness is measured. (Fink, 1993)

The critical assessment, on as objective a basis as possible, of the degree to which entire services or their component parts (e.g. diagnostic tests, treatments, caring procedures) fulfil stated goals. (St Leger et al., 1992)

Evaluation research is the systematic application of social research procedures for assessing the conceptualisation, design, implementation, and utility of social intervention programs. (Rossi and Freeman, 1993)

Any scientifically based activity undertaken to assess the operation and impact of public policies and the action programmes introduced to implement these policies. (Rossi and Wright, 1977)

The purpose of evaluation research is to measure the effects of a programme against the goals it set out to accomplish as a means of contributing to subsequent decision making about the programme and improving future programming. (Weiss, 1977)

The collection, analysis and interpretation of data bearing on the achievements of an organisation's goals and programme objectives. Evaluation usually attempts to measure the extent to which certain outcomes can be validly correlated with inputs and/or outputs. (Phillips et al., 1994)

Any activity that throughout the planning and delivery of innovative programmes enables those involved to make judgements about the starting assumptions, implementation processes and outcomes of the innovation concerned. (Stern, 1993)

Program evaluation is a diligent investigation of a program's characteristics and merits. Its purpose is to provide information on the effectiveness of projects so as to optimise the outcomes, efficiency, and quality of healthcare. (Fink, 1993)

A systematic way of learning from experience and using lessons learnt to improve current activities and promote better planning by careful selection of alternatives for future action. (WHO, 1994 evaluation of 'Health For All', paragraph 108)

Rehabilitation example design

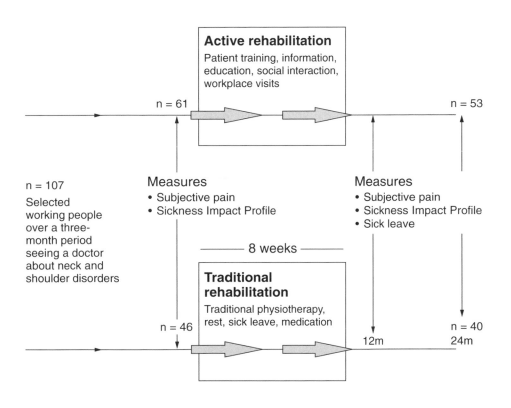

Active rehabilitation
Patient training, information, education, social interaction, workplace visits

n = 61

n = 53

n = 107

Selected working people over a three-month period seeing a doctor about neck and shoulder disorders

Measures
• Subjective pain
• Sickness Impact Profile

Measures
• Subjective pain
• Sickness Impact Profile
• Sick leave

———— 8 weeks ————

Traditional rehabilitation
Traditional physiotherapy, rest, sick leave, medication

n = 46

n = 40

12m

24m

Questions for informants

- Who carried out the activity and what was the activity? (*Describe* the key elements. Any major changes in what you did?)
- Who for? (target group)
- How many? How often? How long?
- Why? (What objectives?)
- How well? (Were objectives met? Would others agree?) (*effectiveness*)
- How *efficient*? (How much was put in, how much came out? What would have given more for the same, quicker, better quality?)
- What difference did it make to the target group? (*Impact* – on others too; any surprises or unintended results?)
- How *relevant and appropriate* for their needs and the needs of those most in need? (Some people more in need not served?)
- How sustainable? (With current funding or a bit more or less?)
- What do you feel proud about? What did you do particularly well?
- What could you have done better and how? (Any mistakes?)
- What would you do differently if you did it again?
- What would you advise a colleague to do and not to do if they were starting?
- Did you do anything which others may not have done?
- What are the strengths and weaknesses?
- What are the main lessons from your experience?
- Any innovations or good practices?
- If others started this elsewhere, what are the important factors or conditions which would help success? What conditions or factors are likely to make it difficult or fail?
- If you were given 10% extra, how would you spend it? If you had to cut 10%, how would you do this?
- What should future programmes like this concentrate on?
- What do you want to say to the people who will read this evaluation?

Appendix 4

Data-gathering plan

1 Evaluation questions or evaluation criteria	2 Data needed to answer this question	3 Sources of data – already collected or collected specially?	4 Method of data collection?	5 How often?	6 Sample?	7 Who is responsible for collecting the data?	8 By when?	9 Method of analysis, presentation and interpretation	10 Why these data will answer the research question (description of input, process or outcome or explanation of cause)
Question 1 Or criteria 1 (e.g. were objectives met?)									
Question 2									
Question 3									
Question 4									
Limitations and how to minimise these and possible problems									

Data for health programme evaluation

The following gives guidance questions for gathering data about a health programme and its performance on the criteria described in Chapter 2.

Programme description and compliance

- Define components of the programme (different interventions for different target populations).
- Define boundaries of the programme (does not cover . . .).
- Define the objectives.
- Describe any major changes over time to the programme, the environment or the targets.
- Describe variations in programme activities from the action plan in the programme proposal.

Achievement of objectives

- What are the objectives of the programme? Are these written down anywhere? Are the objectives measurable and are they measured?
- Level of attainment achieved by the programme? (Or, if objectives are defined, the extent to which the objectives were met?) Ask people for their assessment and proof.
- Were the activities sufficient to meet the agreed objectives?
- Feasibility: were there enough resources to meet the objectives?
- Self-review mechanism: what were the programme procedures for reviewing effectiveness, locally and centrally?
- Issues: the objectives may be unclear or unmeasurable without specifying lower-level objectives; they may be confusing or conflicting where there are too many objectives. (Sort the objectives out using the step model in Appendix 6.)

Outcomes

What would have happened without the programme? What difference did it make and to whom?

Primary targets

- Coverage and quality of service? Who needed the service and did not get it?
- What effects did the programme have on the target populations? (Difference it made, short and long term)
- Were the needs of the targets met?
- Would the resources have had a greater effect if they were used on a subpopulation ('targeting' or 'prioritising')? Has this question been considered and have the ethical issues raised by targeting been considered? What effects on the staff?

Outcomes for other people

- What effects on other people?
- How do we know the programme caused these effects? (What other things could have?)

	Intended	Unintended
Positive		
Negative		

- Issues: getting objective data before and after, reliability of retro-spective subjective views, separating effects of programme from other things, long-term effects.
- Self-review mechanism: what were the programme procedures for reviewing impact, locally and centrally?

Appropriateness

- Appropriateness of the programme: was the programme relevant to the needs of the target groups?
- Appropriateness of the objectives: were the objectives related to the needs of the targets? Should the direction be changed?

- Issues: what are the needs, different views of needs and of the extent to which the programme met them (impact issues)
- Self-review mechanism: what were the programme procedures for reviewing relevance, locally and centrally (i.e. for finding out about needs and adapting the programme to changing needs)?

Efficiency

- What were the inputs (financial (budget headings), staff, supplies, buildings, transport, etc.)?
- What were the outputs (e.g. number of people treated, staff trained)?
- Were any inputs wasted or not used for the intervention programme?
- Could the outputs have been achieved with fewer inputs or in a shorter time or with better quality?
- Issues: compared to what? What level of efficiency is it realistic to expect under the circumstances?
- Self-review mechanism: what were the programme procedures for reviewing efficiency, locally and centrally?

Sustainability

- What are the threats to the programme in the future?
- What is the likelihood of the benefits continuing?
- What would happen if external funding were withdrawn?
- Marginal returns: could many more benefits be produced for a small extra amount of funding or similar benefits be produced with less funding?
- What is the justification for continuing funding or funding a replanned programme?
- Self-review mechanism: what were the programme procedures for planning and ensuring the continuation of the programme, with or without funding?

In some programme evaluations, it may be useful to add the seventh criteria of management performance.

Management performance

Management is an activity which cuts across all the above. Collect data to assess management performance against the following criteria.

- Clarity and appropriateness of programme structure (vertical and lateral co-ordination)
- Quality of planning and budgeting
- Adequacy of systematic review of resource management and replanning (involving cost-benefit assessment of different sub-programmes)
- Adequacy of documentation, monitoring and reporting
- Accuracy and standards of financial accounting
- Performance in supplies management and personnel management
- Compliance with higher-level programme management requirements

Step objectives model

This model serves two purposes. First, when planning a health programme or reform, the model helps to define what is to be done and the steps which will take you to the ultimate long-term aim at the top of the 'step building'. Second, when evaluating an intervention which has many objectives or poorly defined ones, the model shows how to define objectives at different levels of a step hierarchy which shows how objectives build on each other to contribute to the ultimate aim of the intervention.

To 'sort out' the objectives of a health programme or reform you need to:

- list the different objectives (e.g. on 'Post-it' stickers) (LIST)
- cluster those objectives which seem to go together (CLUSTER)
- order the clusters in a hierarchy with the lower level ones below the higher order clusters (LEVELISE)
- take the statements and separate activities from outcomes (you usually have to define outcomes) (SEPARATE)
- finally define the indicators for each objective (INDICATORS).

The model is shown overleaf.

			Ultimate aim
			e.g. HIV is not present in any of the population

		Objective	Indicator
		Reduce the transmission of HIV in the population	e.g. tests of HIV in women giving birth

Step 3

Action	Result	Indicator
e.g. make condoms easily available to the population	e.g. people use condoms for 'safer sex'	e.g. people report using condoms and stocks of condoms are used up

Step 2

Action	Result	Indicator
e.g. provide health education drama events and talks	e.g. people are motivated to do something to protect themselves against HIV	e.g. sample report changes in behaviour and attitudes

Step 1

Action	Result	Indicator
e.g. provide health education information materials	e.g. people are more aware about HIV and AIDS	e.g. 100% of people when questioned are able to explain basic facts about HIV and AIDS

Figure A6.1: Step objectives building model.

Index